A Comprehensive Overview of Endometriosis

Edited by Wei Wu and Rong Ju

Published in London, United Kingdom

A Comprehensive Overview of Endometriosis
http://dx.doi.org/10.5772/intechopen.1000479
Edited by Wei Wu and Rong Ju

Contributors
Ali Emami, Ana Maria Apetrei, Ana Maria Haliciu, Andreea Ioana Pruteanu, Ashish Ashish, Balansama Marah, Daniela Rangel-Santos, Feng Wu, German William Rangel, Gunjan Rai, Haonan Shi, Hongshan Ge, Ioana Pavaleanu, Jing Wei, Jinqi Ma, Kusum Kusum, Lei Chen, Merve Konal, Peihao Wu, Qi Liu, Qinrou Chen, Qiuqin Tang, Raluca Anca Balan, Razvan Socolov, Rong Ju, Royana Singh, Sangeeta Rai, Shivani Mishra, Sia Florence Koroma, Sudhir Diwan, Teodora Ana Balan, Tiberiu Nicolae Poparlan, Tongfei Yang, Tudor Andrei Butureanu, Wei Wu, Xuan Jin, Ying Li, Ziyi Zhang

First published in London, United Kingdom, 2025 by IntechOpen
IntechOpen is the global imprint of INTECHOPEN LIMITED, registered in England and Wales, registration number: 11086078, 167-169 Great Portland Street, London, W1W 5PF, United Kingdom

For EU product safety concerns: IN TECH d.o.o., Prolaz Marije Krucifikse Kozulić 3, 51000 Rijeka, Croatia, info@intechopen.com or visit our website at intechopen.com.

British Library Cataloguing-in-Publication Data
A catalogue record for this book is available from the British Library

A Comprehensive Overview of Endometriosis
Edited by Wei Wu and Rong Ju
p. cm.

This title is part of the Obstetrics and Gynecology Book Series, Volume 7
Topic: Reproductive and Gynecologic Health
Series Editor: Zouhair O. Amarin
Topic Editor: Courtney Marsh

Print ISBN 978-0-85014-733-9
Online ISBN 978-0-85014-732-2
eBook (PDF) ISBN 978-0-85014-734-6
ISSN 3049-706X

IntechOpen Book Series

Obstetrics and Gynecology

Volume 7

Aims and Scope of the Series

Obstetrics and Gynecology field typically covers several subspecialties that include maternal-fetal medicine, gynecologic oncology, reproductive endocrinology and subfertility, urogynecology and female pelvic reconstructive surgery, critical care medicine, complex family planning, pediatric and adolescent gynecology, menopausal and geriatric gynecology, and minimally invasive gynecologic surgery.
Apart from being diverse, obstetrics and gynecology is a challenging and demanding specialty. It combines medical and surgical skills.
The sequence of books in this series will have certain characteristics in common that will be recognized as part of the same informative multi-volume book programme.

Meet the Series Editor

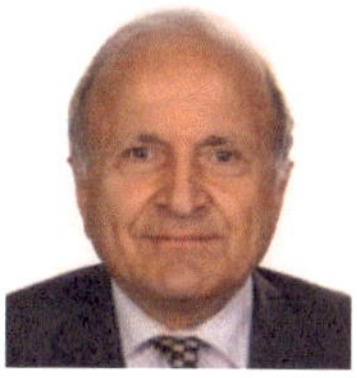

Zouhair Amarin is a Professor of Obstetrics and Gynaecology at the Jordan University of Science and Technology. He was previously a lecturer at the University of Glasgow, Scotland, a senior lecturer at the University of Nottingham, England, and the dean of the Faculty of Medicine at Mutah University, Jordan. Professor Amarin is a fellow of the Royal College of Obstetricians and Gynaecologists, and the Faculty of Public Health, London. He holds master's degrees in medical science and medical education. He is a pioneer in IVF and was the first in the world to develop microsurgical epididymis sperm aspiration for clinical use. He also discovered a surgical procedure for critical ovarian hyperstimulation syndrome. Professor Amarin has edited books, authored book chapters, and published more than 130 papers. He is the recipient of eight awards.

Meet the Volume Editors

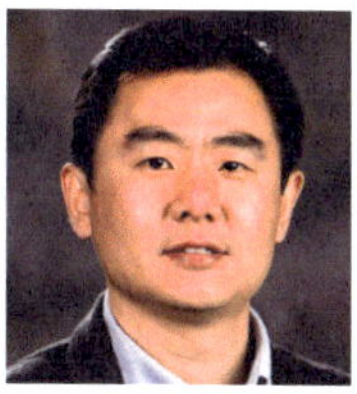

Dr. Wei Wu is a Professor at the School of Public Health and the Vice Dean of the School of International Education at Nanjing Medical University, China. He has served as a guest researcher at the National Institute of Environmental Health Sciences (NIEHS). Dr. Wu is an active member of various national and international societies in the fields of human reproduction and toxicology, and he has received numerous awards from prestigious organizations for the originality and quality of his research projects. Dr. Wu has authored 90 peer-reviewed papers in international journals, achieving an H-index of 30. In addition to his research contributions, he has edited nine books and contributed to ten other volumes. He holds 20 patents and has organized six international conferences. Furthermore, he serves as a reviewer for 112 academic journals.

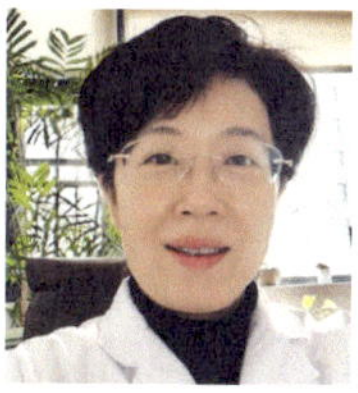

Dr. Rong Ju is the Vice Director of Nanjing Jiangning Hospital. She has been engaged in clinical and teaching in obstetrics and gynecology for over 20 years, focusing on research in gynecological reproductive endocrinology, endometriosis, infectious diseases, and hospital management. Dr. Ju is an active member of various societies in the fields of human reproduction, endocrinology, obstetrics and gynecology, and developmental biology. She has presided over 10 research projects and published over 30 papers.

Contents

Preface

Endometriosis is a complex and often misunderstood gynecological condition that presents significant challenges for medical professionals and the millions of women affected globally. As the editor of this comprehensive volume, I am pleased to present a carefully curated collection of chapters that explore the intricate nature of endometriosis, covering aspects from its pathogenesis and diagnosis to treatment options and the broader implications for patients' lives.

Chapter 1 comprehensively reviews the diverse symptoms of endometriosis, covering gastrointestinal, urogenital, thoracic, cutaneous, and neurological manifestations. It highlights diagnostic challenges and their impact on quality of life, emphasizing the need for accurate diagnostic tools and personalized treatment strategies.

Chapter 2 explores endometriosis-associated ovarian carcinoma (EAOC), examining its epidemiological links, molecular mechanisms, and clinical implications. It highlights risk factors, pathological characteristics, and the distinct subtypes of EAOC, emphasizing the importance of early detection and targeted treatments.

Chapter 3 offers a comprehensive overview of medical treatments for endometriosis, covering hormonal therapies, non-hormonal treatments, emerging approaches, and lifestyle modifications. It emphasizes personalized treatment strategies and the importance of patient education for long-term management.

Chapter 4 comprehensively reviews pain management strategies for women with endometriosis, covering pharmacological treatments, interventional techniques, and adjuvant therapies. This comprehensive review underscores the need to integrate different treatment modalities to address the diverse symptoms and challenges these patients face, ensuring a more holistic and effective pain management.

Chapter 5 comprehensively reviews recent advances in endometriosis research, from genetic factors and environmental influences to emerging technologies and personalized medicine approaches.

Chapter 6 explores the role of environmental exposures and epigenetic factors in endometriosis, discussing how these elements influence disease development and potential applications in diagnosis and treatment.

Throughout the writing process, I have had the honor of collaborating with a dedicated team of co-editors and contributors, each offering their unique expertise and perspectives. Their combined efforts have been crucial in producing a comprehensive and authoritative resource on endometriosis. I would like to thank Mrs. Maja Bozicevic at IntechOpen for her strong support from the inception to the completion of this book. The completion of this book was made possible with the support of the

Noncommunicable Chronic Diseases-National Science and Technology Major Project (2023ZD0507401).

In conclusion, *A Comprehensive Overview of Endometriosis* is designed to be a valuable resource for medical professionals, researchers, and patients. We hope the information in this work will enhance understanding of endometriosis, encourage further research, and ultimately improve diagnosis, treatment, and support for individuals affected by this complex condition.

Wei Wu
School of Public Health,
Nanjing Medical University,
China

Rong Ju
The Affiliated Jiangning Hospital of Nanjing Medical University,
Nanjing Medical University,
China

Chapter 1

Decoding Endometriosis: A Comprehensive Guide to Understanding Symptoms and Impacts

Ali Emami

Abstract

Up to 10% of all women suffer with endometriosis, a chronic inflammatory gynecological condition, that is dependent on estrogen. This prevalence rises to 30–50% among women who experience infertility and/or severe pelvic pain. Endometriosis is a disease that is remarkably underdiagnosed and undertreated due to a lack of exact knowledge about it. It takes an unreasonable amount of time (8–12 years) between the onset of symptoms and a conclusive diagnosis. This is due to the fact that the majority of the symptoms are non-specific and there are no non-invasive diagnostic procedures that can offer a conclusive diagnosis. These days, assessing all symptoms and indicators that may lead us to question the presence of endometriosis is crucial. We will investigate all symptoms of this disorder in this chapter.

Keywords: endometriosis, symptoms, signs, fatigue, chronic pelvic pain

1. Introduction

Endometriosis is a persistent inflammatory, estrogen-dependent disorder characterized by the growth of endometrial-like tissue outside the uterine cavity [1, 2]. This condition affects an estimated 175 million women of reproductive age worldwide [3].

Endometriosis is estimated to affect one in ten Australian women of reproductive age, incurring direct medical and surgical costs exceeding $6 billion annually for women over 18 years old [4]. The definitive diagnosis of endometriosis necessitates laparoscopy and histopathology [5]. For many women, the interval between the onset of symptoms and diagnosis can exceed 8 years. Consequently, there is significant interest in identifying clinical features that could predict the presence of endometriosis and reduce the delay in commencing active treatment [6].

Endometriosis is influenced by several known risk factors, including early menarche, late menopause, short menstrual cycles, low body mass index (BMI), and low parity [7, 8]. The etiopathogenesis of endometriosis remains not fully understood.

Potential contributing factors include uterine hyperperistalsis and hyperestrogenism, alongside genetic factors, the implantation theory, and cellular metaplasia [9, 10].

It is widely believed that the extent of anatomical distortion caused by adhesions and fibrosis from endometriosis correlates with higher incidences of infertility. Additionally, soluble factors such as inflammation, oxidative stress, hormonal abnormalities, and immune dysregulation play significant roles in infertility among endometriosis patients. Chronic wounds, including those from endometriosis, diabetic foot ulcers, and other non-healing conditions, undergo recurrent tissue damage and repair cycles [11, 12]. In endometriosis, fibrosis is induced by inflammatory responses, leading to processes like epithelial-mesenchymal transition (EMT), fibroblast-myofibroblast transdifferentiation (FMT), and smooth muscle metaplasia (SMM), perpetuating the cycle of wound healing and tissue remodeling [13, 14].

The classical clinical presentation of endometriosis includes dysmenorrhea, dyspareunia, infertility, and menstrual cycle-related lower abdominal pain. These symptoms can guide clinicians toward the correct diagnosis [15, 16]. However, in Germany, endometriosis is often diagnosed with a delay of up to 10 years, primarily due to misdiagnosis. This issue is particularly pronounced in cases of extragenital endometriosis (EE), which affects approximately 9% of women with endometriosis [17].

EE cases are frequently first presented to non-gynecological specialties, leading to delayed diagnosis and chronic pain, which can dysregulate the nervous system and cause abnormal pain patterns. This necessitates a more complex differential diagnosis process, having significant physical, psychological, and social impacts. Early recognition and proper treatment initiation are crucial [18, 19]. Recent research has concentrated on identifying reliable biomarkers for endometriosis, encompassing a wide range of indicators. These include immunologic markers such as immune cells, antibodies, and cytokines, as well as genetic and biochemical markers like microRNAs, long non-coding RNAs (lncRNAs), circulating and mitochondrial nucleic acids. Additionally, some hormones, glycoproteins, and signaling molecules have also been identified as potential biomarkers [20, 21].

The diagnostic process begins with a thorough clinical history, exploring whether symptoms correlate with menstrual cycle phases. Clinical examination includes speculum examination, palpation (including rectovaginal palpation), transvaginal ultrasound, and renal ultrasound. Diagnostic laparoscopy is the gold standard for histological confirmation [22].

Identifying superficial diseases, peritoneal lesions, or early/mild deep endometriosis through imaging techniques remains challenging, which suggests that a negative result does not exclude the presence of endometriosis. However, transvaginal sonography (TVS) and magnetic resonance imaging (MRI) are effective for detecting more advanced stages of the condition. Severe endometriosis is characterized by extensive adhesions to surrounding organs, such as significant inflammatory adhesions between ovarian endometrioma and the rectum. TVS is particularly valuable for diagnosing adhesions via dynamic manipulation of pelvic organs, where reduced ovarian mobility and limited sliding between the posterior uterine serosa and bowel indicate adhesion presence [23, 24].

Women displaying TVS signs of ovarian endometriomas exhibit higher levels of ovarian immobility than those without these features, with a sensitivity and specificity of 89% and 90%, respectively [25, 26]. The capacity of MRI to detect adhesions and obliteration of the pouch of Douglas is similar to that of dynamic TVS, which diminishes the necessity for routine MRI following TVS. Thus, the diagnostic precision of dynamic TVS rivals may even surpass, that of routine MRI, although MRI offers greater objectivity and reproducibility. Both TVS and MRI serve as critical tools in assessing the severity of endometriosis, particularly in identifying adhesions, and may contribute to establishing a classification for endometriosis-associated pain. Conversely, a major challenge remains unresolved regarding endometriosis-related infertility, as imaging techniques focused on structural anomalies may not correlate with the progression of infertility severity [25, 27, 28].

Due to the chronic nature of endometriosis, a long-term, personalized treatment plan is essential, encompassing both conservative (symptomatic and hormonal) and surgical treatments, with the potential integration of complementary medicine. Surgical indications include organ destruction, differential diagnosis for sterility, and persistent pain, with a goal of complete laparoscopic resection where possible. Studies have not demonstrated a clear advantage of surgical treatment over pharmacotherapy for endometriosis-associated pain. Pharmacotherapy aims to achieve secondary amenorrhea, with dienogest being the first-line drug. Other options include combined oral contraceptives, gonadotropin-releasing hormone (GnRH) analogs, and local progestins. In order to lower the likelihood of recurrence, hormonal therapy is advised following surgery, unless pregnancy is urgently wanted [9].

2. Gastrointestinal symptoms

Bowel endometriosis is defined by the presence of endometriotic lesions that infiltrate at least the muscular layer of the intestinal wall [29]. Superficial endometriotic lesions, which only penetrate the intestinal serosa, should not be classified as bowel endometriosis and are generally asymptomatic. This condition is estimated to affect between 5% and 25% of patients diagnosed surgically with endometriosis [30]. The majority of bowel endometriotic nodules are located at the rectosigmoid junction and rectum (65.7%); however, lesions can also be noted in the sigmoid colon (17.4%), caecum and ileocecal junction (4.1%), appendix (6.4%), and omentum (1.7%) [31].

Patients with bowel endometriosis typically experience pain and intestinal symptoms. The pain can be attributed to the intestinal nodules as well as other deep endometriotic nodules, such as those found in the rectovaginal septum, uterosacral ligaments, and parametrium, which are often associated with intestinal lesions. In addition, the location, size, and degree of intestinal lumen stenosis of bowel nodules might result in a range of intestinal symptoms (**Figures 1** and **2**) [32].

Patients with rectosigmoid endometriosis may present with a range of intestinal symptoms, including dyschezia, cyclic bowel alterations, abdominal cramping, a sensation of incomplete evacuation, stool fragmentation, the passage of mucus with stools, and rectal bleeding [33].

The most common complaints among patients included constipation (40%), a feeling of incomplete evacuation (36%), and stool fragmentation (52%). The severity of dyschezia, as measured on a 10-point visual analog scale, averaged 7.1. Patients with deep endometriosis infiltrating the rectum were more likely to experience cyclic defecation pain (67.9%) and cyclic constipation (54.7%), and they also exhibited a significantly longer time to evacuate stools. However, these symptoms were also prevalent in other groups studied, with 38.1% and 33.3% for the superficial endometriosis group, and 42.9% and 26.2% for the group with deep endometriosis sparing the rectum, respectively. Women with rectal endometriosis were also more prone to appetite disorders [34].

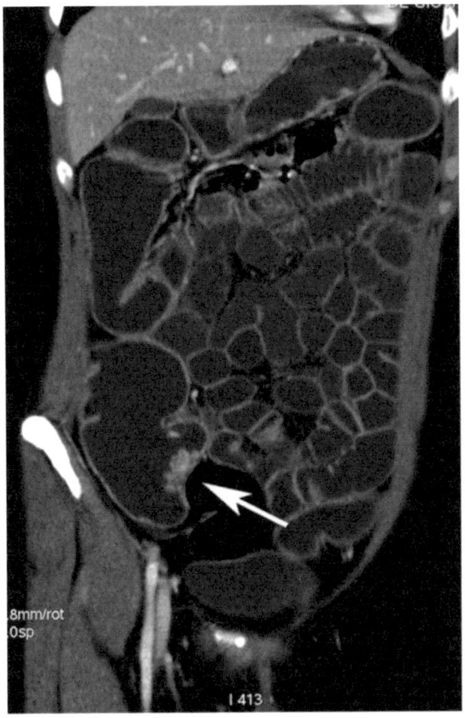

Figure 1.
Cecal endometriotic nodule (arrow) [32].

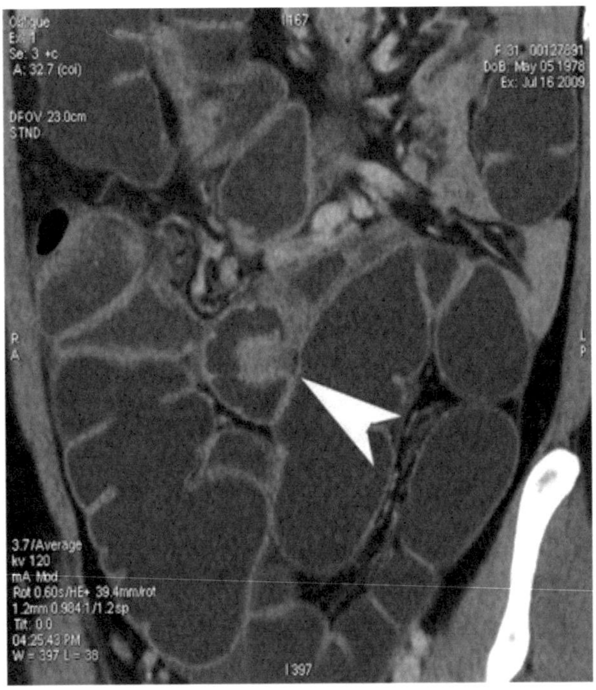

Figure 2.
Ileal endometriotic nodule (arrowhead) [32].

The pain and intestinal symptoms associated with rectosigmoid endometriosis are nonspecific, often leading to diagnostic challenges. Prior to receiving a definitive diagnosis, patients with endometriosis are frequently misdiagnosed with conditions such as irritable bowel syndrome (IBS). An Australian study examined the intestinal symptoms of patients with endometriosis, highlighting these diagnostic complexities [35].

Ileocecal endometriosis may manifest as intestinal obstruction, intussusception, or ileocecal perforation, leading to symptoms such as intestinal cramps, vomiting, abdominal distention, and catamenial subocclusion [36–39]. In some cases, ileocecal endometriosis can cause nonspecific symptoms that resemble those of intestinal malignancies or Crohn's disease. While magnetic resonance imaging and computed tomography may detect an ileocecal mass, they do not always conclusively indicate endometriosis [32].

Double-contrast barium enema is ineffective at detecting small extraluminal lesions. Occasionally, isolated ileocecal endometriosis may be asymptomatic and can present as a submucosal polyp during screening colonoscopy [40]. There have been documented cases of ileocecal perforation related to endometriosis occurring during pregnancy and postpartum. Due to the high vascularization of ectopic endometriotic tissue, ileocolic perforation during pregnancy can lead to significant intraperitoneal hemorrhage [41, 42].

Appendiceal endometriosis occurs in approximately 2.6% of patients undergoing surgery for endometriosis [43]. The diagnosis of appendiceal endometriosis is often made incidentally during surgery for endometriosis-related pain, without preoperative suspicion of its presence on the appendix. However, in some patients, gross alterations of the appendix may necessitate a selective appendectomy [44].

Appendiceal endometriosis can mimic acute appendicitis, presenting with symptoms such as fever, right lower quadrant pain, nausea, and vomiting, and signs such as pain at McBurney's point [45]. There have been reports of appendiceal perforation due to endometriosis [46]. The acute inflammation is often a result of endometriosis causing partial or complete occlusion of the appendiceal lumen. Rarely, endometriosis can result in appendiceal intussusception as well [47].

3. Urogenital symptoms

Urogenital tract endometriosis (UGE) is the second most common form of EE, primarily affecting the bladder (over 85% of cases) and, less frequently, the ureters (10%), kidneys (4%), and urethra (2%) [48].

It typically occurs in women aged 30 to 45 years, with prior pelvic surgery considered a risk factor. Familial aggregation has also been reported [49]. UGE can be asymptomatic in up to 50% of cases, though it can lead to significant complications such as complete loss of kidney function in severe cases of ureteral endometriosis [50].

Bladder endometriosis may present with dysuria, recurrent urinary tract infections, hematuria, irritable bladder symptoms, vesical tenesmus, and incontinence. About 40% of women with bladder endometriosis experience perimenstrual symptoms. Ureteral endometriosis, which affects about 15% of patients, may present with costovertebral angle pain or hematuria [48, 51, 52].

Surgery is advised for bladder endometriosis lesions, and hydronephrosis is a clear sign that surgery is necessary. Re-implantation and ureteral excision are further treatment options, with ureterolysis being successful in 86.7% of cases [51].

4. Thoracic symptoms

Thoracic endometriosis (TE) is a rare form of endometriosis affecting the diaphragm (**Figure 3**) (44.5%), pleura (12.7%), and lungs (4.5%), often involving multiple structures simultaneously. Genital endometriosis coexists in 53–84% of TE cases. TE typically presents around the ages of 30 to 34, about 5 years later than genital endometriosis [18, 53].

Symptoms include menstrual cycle-related, usually right-sided pain in the thoracic, scapular, or shoulder region, and catamenial pneumothorax [18]. Diagnosis involves correlating symptoms with menstruation and diagnostic radiology, with MRI being the preferred modality [54].

Bronchoscopy is useful in cases of hemoptysis to rule out other conditions. Histological confirmation is necessary for a definitive diagnosis. Surgical management often involves a two-stage approach followed by medical treatment, with video-assisted thoracoscopic surgery (VATS) and, in some cases, laparoscopy [54–56].

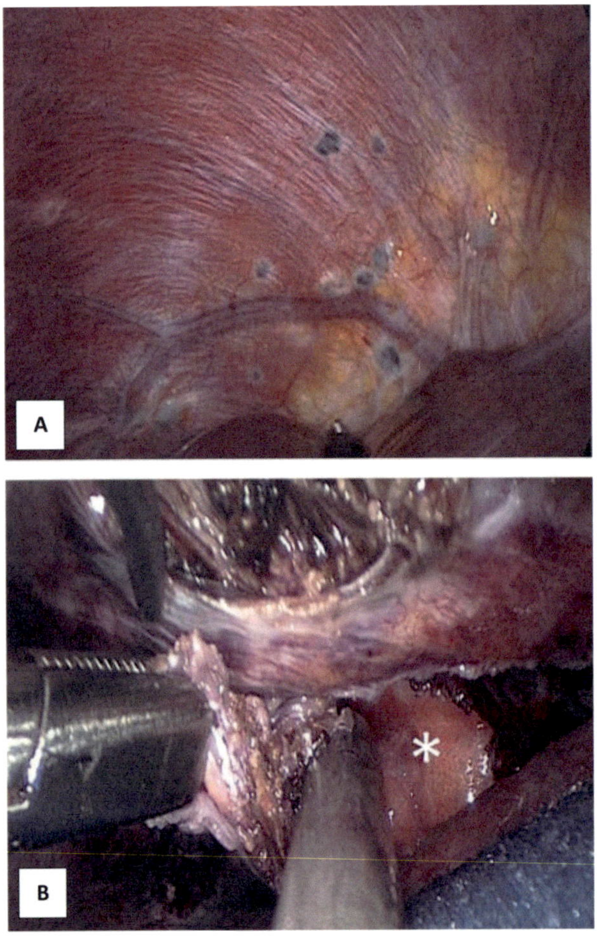

Figure 3.
Multiple diaphragmatic endometriosis (the star in picture B is the lung tissue) [22].

5. Skin symptoms

Cutaneous scar endometriosis can occur following cesarean delivery, hysterectomy, or laparoscopy, presenting as nodules in the epifascial tissue. This pathology affects less than 1% of women with endometriosis and can be easily excised. Overall, endometriosis requires a comprehensive diagnostic and treatment approach, tailored to the individual patient's needs and clinical presentation [22, 57].

6. Neurology symptoms

Nerve involvement, particularly of the sacral plexus, including the sciatic nerve, is a rare manifestation of EE. Approximately 34% of patients exhibit nerve involvement without peritoneal lesions. The etiology may involve the development of endometriosis lesions from undifferentiated cells within the nerve [58].

Symptoms include cyclic (perimenstrual) sciatica, and prolonged untreated conditions may lead to constant pain and neurological deficits. MRI is the diagnostic tool of choice, with ultrasonography as an alternative. Successful drug treatments are rare, and surgical excision of parametrial and peritoneal lesions significantly improves quality of life and pain symptoms [58, 59].

7. Conclusions

This comprehensive review of endometriosis symptoms highlights the multifaceted nature of the disease, which presents with a wide range of symptoms affecting various systems including gastrointestinal, urogenital, thoracic, cutaneous, and neurological. Despite its prevalence, endometriosis remains underdiagnosed and undertreated, with significant delays in diagnosis that can exacerbate patient suffering and complicate treatment.

Key findings from this review include the recognition of bowel endometriosis as a significant source of gastrointestinal symptoms, often misdiagnosed as irritable bowel syndrome (IBS). Similarly, urogenital and thoracic endometriosis present with symptoms that are frequently mistaken for other conditions, further complicating timely diagnosis. The review also emphasizes the importance of considering less common manifestations of the disease, such as nerve involvement and cutaneous scar endometriosis, which, though rare, can significantly impact the quality of life.

The challenges in diagnosing endometriosis underscore the need for greater awareness among healthcare providers and the development of more accurate and less invasive diagnostic tools. Additionally, given the chronic nature of endometriosis, long-term management strategies that integrate both medical and surgical approaches are essential.

Future research should focus on improving diagnostic methodologies, including the development of non-invasive tests, and exploring the pathophysiological mechanisms underlying the diverse presentations of the disease. Furthermore, clinical practice would benefit from a multidisciplinary approach to treatment, tailored to the individual symptoms and needs of patients, to optimize outcomes and improve the quality of life for those affected by endometriosis.

Acknowledgements

Hereby, we would like to thank the Clinical Research Development Center of Kowsar Hospital and the Student Research Committee of Qazvin University of Medical Sciences, Qazvin, Iran.

The author acknowledges the use of ChatGPT by OpenAI and the Grammarly Web site for editing the grammar and punctuation. The authors have not declared a specific grant for this research from any funding agency.

Conflict of interest

The author declared no conflict of interest.

Author details

Ali Emami
Qazvin University of Medical Sciences, Qazvin, Iran

*Address all correspondence to: aliiemamii74@gmail.com

References

[1] Horne AW, Missmer SA. Pathophysiology, diagnosis, and management of endometriosis. BMJ. 2022;**379**:2-3

[2] Reis FM, Petraglia F, Taylor RN. Endometriosis: Hormone regulation and clinical consequences of chemotaxis and apoptosis. Human Reproduction Update. 2013;**19**(4):406-418

[3] Adamson GD, Pasta DJ. Endometriosis fertility index: The new, validated endometriosis staging system. Fertility and Sterility. 2010;**94**(5):1609-1615

[4] Bush D, Evans S, Vancaille T. The $6 Billion Woman and the $600 Million Girl. The Pelvic Pain report. Melbourne: Pain Australia and the Faculty of Pain medicine; 2011

[5] Dunselman G, Vermeulen N, Becker C, Calhaz-Jorge C, D'hooghe T, De Bie B, et al. ESHRE guideline: Management of women with endometriosis. Human Reproduction. 2014;**29**(3):400-412

[6] Agarwal SK, Chapron C, Giudice LC, Laufer MR, Leyland N, Missmer SA, et al. Clinical diagnosis of endometriosis: A call to action. American Journal of Obstetrics and Gynecology. 2019;**220**(4):354.e351-354.e312

[7] Shafrir AL, Farland L, Shah D, Harris H, Kvaskoff M, Zondervan K, et al. Risk for and consequences of endometriosis: A critical epidemiologic review. Best Practice & Research. Clinical Obstetrics & Gynaecology. 2018;**51**:1-15

[8] Zhang Y, Ma N-Y. Environmental risk factors for endometriosis: An umbrella review of a meta-analysis of 354 observational studies with over 5 million populations. Frontiers in Medicine. 2021;**8**:680833

[9] Burghaus S, Schaefer SD, Beckmann MW, Brandes I, Bruenahl C, Chvatal R, et al. Diagnosis and treatment of endometriosis. Guideline of the DGGG, SGGG and OEGGG (S2k Level, AWMF registry number 015/045, august 2020). Geburtshilfe und Frauenheilkunde. 2021;**81**(04):422-446

[10] Signorile PG, Viceconte R, Baldi A. New insights in pathogenesis of endometriosis. Frontiers in Medicine. 2022;**9**:879015

[11] Augoulea A, Mastorakos G, Lambrinoudaki I, Christodoulakos G, Creatsas G. The role of the oxidative-stress in the endometriosis-related infertility. Gynecological Endocrinology. 2009;**25**(2):75-81

[12] Jackson L, Schisterman E, Dey-Rao R, Browne R, Armstrong D. Oxidative stress and endometriosis. Human Reproduction. 2005;**20**(7):2014-2020

[13] Capobianco A, Cottone L, Monno A, Manfredi AA, Rovere-Querini P. The peritoneum: Healing, immunity, and diseases. The Journal of Pathology. 2017;**243**(2):137-147

[14] Guo S-W, Ding D, Shen M, Liu X. Dating endometriotic ovarian cysts based on the content of cyst fluid and its potential clinical implications. Reproductive Sciences. 2015;**22**(7):873-883

[15] Ali O, Amso NN. Endometriosis: Clinical manifestation and differential diagnosis. In: Endometriosis. Taylor & Francis, CRC Press; 2022. pp. 7-26

[16] Coutureau J, Mandoul C, Verheyden C, Millet I, Taourel P. Acute abdominal pain in women of reproductive age: Keys to suggest a complication of endometriosis. Insights Into Imaging. 2023;**14**(1):94

[17] Hudelist G, Fritzer N, Thomas A, Niehues C, Oppelt P, Haas D, et al. Diagnostic delay for endometriosis in Austria and Germany: Causes and possible consequences. Human Reproduction. 2012;**27**(12):3412-3416

[18] Andres MP, Arcoverde FV, Souza CC, Fernandes LFC, Abrao MS, Kho RM. Extrapelvic endometriosis: A systematic review. Journal of Minimally Invasive Gynecology. 2020;**27**(2):373-389

[19] Cromeens MG, Carey ET, Robinson WR, Knafl K, Thoyre S. Timing, delays and pathways to diagnosis of endometriosis: A scoping review protocol. BMJ Open. 2021;**11**(6):e049390

[20] Mahini SM, Younesi M, Mortazavi G, Samare-Najaf M, Azadbakht MK, Jamali N. Non-invasive diagnosis of endometriosis: Immunologic and genetic markers. Clinica Chimica Acta. 2023;**538**:70-86

[21] Samare-Najaf M, Razavinasab SA, Samareh A, Jamali N. Omics-based novel strategies in the diagnosis of endometriosis. Critical Reviews in Clinical Laboratory Sciences. 2024;**61**(3):205-225

[22] Lukac S, Schmid M, Pfister K, Janni W, Schäffler H, Dayan D. Extragenital endometriosis in the differential diagnosis of non-gynecological diseases. Deutsches Ärzteblatt International. 2022;**119**(20):361

[23] Holland T, Yazbek J, Cutner A, Saridogan E, Hoo W, Jurkovic D. Value of transvaginal ultrasound in assessing severity of pelvic endometriosis. Ultrasound in Obstetrics and Gynecology. 2010;**36**(2):241-248

[24] Zanardi R, Del Frate C, Zuiani C, Bazzocchi M. Staging of pelvic endometriosis based on MRI findings versus laparoscopic classification according to the American Fertility Society. Abdominal Imaging. 2003;**28**:733-742

[25] Gerges B, Lu C, Reid S, Chou D, Chang T, Condous G. Sonographic evaluation of immobility of normal and endometriotic ovary in detection of deep endometriosis. Ultrasound in Obstetrics & Gynecology. 2017;**49**(6):793-798

[26] Guerriero S, Ajossa S, Garau N, Alcazar JL, Mais V, Melis GB. Diagnosis of pelvic adhesions in patients with endometrioma: The role of transvaginal ultrasonography. Fertility and Sterility. 2010;**94**(2):742-746

[27] Ichikawa M, Akira S, Kaseki H, Watanabe K, Ono S, Takeshita T. Accuracy and clinical value of an adhesion scoring system: A preoperative diagnostic method using transvaginal ultrasonography for endometriotic adhesion. Journal of Obstetrics and Gynaecology Research. 2020;**46**(3):466-478

[28] Wilde R, Alvarez J, Brölmann H, Campo R, Cheong Y, Lundorff P, et al. Adhesions and endometriosis: Challenges in subfertility management. Archives of Gynecology and Obstetrics. 2016;**2**(294):299-301

[29] Remorgida V, Ferrero S, Fulcheri E, Ragni N, Martin DC. Bowel endometriosis: Presentation, diagnosis, and treatment. Obstetrical & Gynecological Survey. 2007;**62**(7):461-470

[30] Audebert A, Petousis S, Margioula-Siarkou C, Ravanos K, Prapas N, Prapas Y. Anatomic distribution of endometriosis: A reappraisal based on series of 1101 patients. European Journal of Obstetrics & Gynecology and Reproductive Biology. 2018;**230**:36-40

[31] Chapron C, Chopin N, Borghese B, Foulot H, Dousset B, Vacher-Lavenu MC, et al. Deeply infiltrating endometriosis: Pathogenetic implications of the anatomical distribution. Human Reproduction. 2006;**21**(7):1839-1845

[32] Ferrero S, Moioli M, Dodero D, Barra F. Symptoms of bowel endometriosis. In: Clinical Management of Bowel Endometriosis: From Diagnosis to Treatment. Cham: Springer; 2020. pp. 33-39

[33] Abrao MS, Petraglia F, Falcone T, Keckstein J, Osuga Y, Chapron C. Deep endometriosis infiltrating the recto-sigmoid: Critical factors to consider before management. Human Reproduction Update. 2015;**21**(3):329-339

[34] Roman H, Ness J, Suciu N, Bridoux V, Gourcerol G, Leroi AM, et al. Are digestive symptoms in women presenting with pelvic endometriosis specific to lesion localizations? A preliminary prospective study. Human Reproduction. 2012;**27**(12):3440-3449

[35] Maroun P, Cooper MJ, Reid GD, Keirse MJ. Relevance of gastrointestinal symptoms in endometriosis. Australian and New Zealand Journal of Obstetrics and Gynaecology. 2009;**49**(4):411-414

[36] Arata R, Takakura Y, Ikeda S, Itamoto T. A case of ileus caused by ileal endometriosis with lymph node involvement. International Journal of Surgery Case Reports. 2019;**54**:90-94

[37] Marques-Ruiz A, Camara-Baena S, Sanchez-Ramos Y. A new reported case of ileocecal infiltrative endometriosis, a disease which is probably underdiagnosed. Revista Espanola de Enfermadades Digestivas (REED). 2018;**110**(12):835-837

[38] Guerra Veloz MF, Gómez Rodríguez BJ, Benallal DC. Ileocecal endometriosis as an infrequent cause of intussusception. Revista Espanola de Enfermedades Digestivas: Organo Oficial de la Sociedad Espanola de Patologia Digestiva. 2018;**110**(2):129-129

[39] Rodriguez-Lopez M, Bailon-Cuadrado M, Tejero-Pintor F, Choolani E, Fernandez-Perez G, Tapia-Herrero A. Ileocecal intussusception extending to left colon due to endometriosis. The Annals of The Royal College of Surgeons of England. 2018;**100**(3):e62-e63

[40] James O, Williams GL. Prolapsing mass in the caecum: Learning point for the colonoscopist. BMJ Case Reports. 2019;**12**(4):1-2

[41] Beamish RE, Aslam R, Gilbert JM. Postpartum caecal perforation due to endometriosis. JRSM Short Reports. 2010;**1**(7):1-3

[42] Nishikawa A, Kondoh E, Hamanishi J, Yamaguchi K, Ueda A, Sato Y, et al. Ileal perforation and massive intestinal haemorrhage from endometriosis in pregnancy: Case report and literature review. European Journal of Obstetrics & Gynecology and Reproductive Biology. 2013;**170**(1):20-24

[43] Mabrouk M, Raimondo D, Mastronardi M, Raimondo I, Del Forno S, Arena A, et al. Endometriosis of the appendix: When to predict and how to manage—A multivariate analysis of 1935 endometriosis cases. Journal

of Minimally Invasive Gynecology. 2020;**27**(1):100-106

[44] Moulder JK, Siedhoff MT, Melvin KL, Jarvis EG, Hobbs KA, Garrett J. Risk of appendiceal endometriosis among women with deep-infiltrating endometriosis. International Journal of Gynecology & Obstetrics. 2017;**139**(2):149-154

[45] John BS, Snider A, Kellermier H, Minhas S, Nottingham J. Endometriosis of the appendix presenting as acute appendicitis with unusual appearance. International Journal of Surgery Case Reports. 2018;**53**:211-213

[46] Akbulut S, Dursun P, Kocbiyik A, Harman A, Sevmis S. Appendiceal endometriosis presenting as perforated appendicitis: Report of a case and review of the literature. Archives of Gynecology and Obstetrics. 2009;**280**:495-497

[47] Dickson-Lowe RA, Ibrahim S, Munthali L, Hasan F. Intussusception of the vermiform appendix. Case Reports. 2015;**2015**:bcr2014207584

[48] Leonardi M, Espada M, Kho RM, Magrina JF, Millischer A-E, Savelli L, et al. Endometriosis and the urinary tract: From diagnosis to surgical treatment. Diagnostics. 2020;**10**(10):771

[49] Charatsi D, Koukoura O, Ntavela IG, Chintziou F, Gkorila G, Tsagkoulis M, et al. Gastrointestinal and urinary tract endometriosis: A review on the commonest locations of extrapelvic endometriosis. Advances in Medicine. 2018;**2018**(1):3461209

[50] Bretón SA, Carrasco AL, Gutiérrez AH, González RR, de Santiago García J. Complete loss of unilateral renal function secondary to endometriosis: A report of three cases. European Journal of Obstetrics & Gynecology and Reproductive Biology. 2013;**171**(1):132-137

[51] Cavaco-Gomes J, Martinho M, Gilabert-Aguilar J, Gilabert-Estélles J. Laparoscopic management of ureteral endometriosis: A systematic review. European Journal of Obstetrics & Gynecology and Reproductive Biology. 2017;**210**:94-101

[52] Leone Roberti Maggiore U, Ferrero S, Salvatore S. Urinary incontinence and bladder endometriosis: Conservative management. International Urogynecology Journal. 2015;**26**:159-162

[53] Joseph J, Sahn SA. Thoracic endometriosis syndrome: New observations from an analysis of 110 cases. The American Journal of Medicine. 1996;**100**(2):164-170

[54] Rousset P, Gregory J, Rousset-Jablonski C, Hugon-Rodin J, Regnard J-F, Chapron C, et al. MR diagnosis of diaphragmatic endometriosis. European Radiology. 2016;**26**:3968-3977

[55] Korom S, Canyurt H, Missbach A, Schneiter D, Kurrer MO, Haller U, et al. Catamenial pneumothorax revisited: Clinical approach and systematic review of the literature. The Journal of Thoracic and Cardiovascular Surgery. 2004;**128**(4):502-508

[56] Tulandi T, Sirois C, Sabban H, Cohen A, Murji A, Singh SS, et al. Relationship between catamenial pneumothorax or non-catamenial pneumothorax and endometriosis. Journal of Minimally Invasive Gynecology. 2018;**25**(3):480-483

[57] Danielpour PJ, Layke JC, Durie N, Glickman LT. Scar endometriosis—A rare cause for a painful scar: A case

report and review of the literature. Canadian Journal of Plastic Surgery. 2010;**18**(1):19-20

[58] Siquara De Sousa AC, Capek S, Amrami KK, Spinner RJ. Neural involvement in endometriosis: Review of anatomic distribution and mechanisms. Clinical Anatomy. 2015;**28**(8):1029-1038

[59] Niro J, Fournier M, Oberlin C, Le Tohic A, Panel P. Endometriotic lesions of the lower troncular nerves. Gynécologie, Obstétrique & Fertilité. 2014;**42**(10):702-705

Chapter 2

Endometriosis-Associated Ovarian Carcinoma

Ioana Pavaleanu, Teodora Ana Balan,
Tiberiu Nicolae Poparlan, Ana Maria Haliciu,
Tudor Andrei Butureanu, Ana Maria Apetrei, Razvan Socolov,
Andreea Ioana Pruteanu and Raluca Anca Balan

Abstract

The link between endometriosis and ovarian carcinoma has been recognized early on, initially termed endometriosis-associated ovarian carcinoma and subsequently referred to as endometriosis-associated ovarian carcinoma (EAOC). The relationship between endometriosis and cancer is well supported by epidemiological evidence, highlighting common risk factors. Two potential mechanisms have been proposed: one involving the direct malignant transformation of endometriotic lesions, and the other suggesting a shared origin in precursor mechanisms or risk factors, followed by distinct molecular pathways. This chapter explores the epidemiological links, molecular mechanisms, and clinical implications of endometriosis-associated ovarian carcinoma, highlighting its distinct subtypes and risk factors.

Keywords: endometriosis, endometriosis-associated ovarian carcinoma, endometriosis-related ovarian neoplasm, ovarian malignancy, malignant transformation

1. Introduction

Endometriosis is a gynecological entity characterized by the presence of ectopic endometrium outside the uterus, in a multitude of locations, mainly in ovary (67%), followed by anterior and posterior cul de sac, uterosacral ligaments, posterior broad ligaments, fallopian tubes, round ligaments, and sigmoid colon or appendix [1]. Other less frequent locations are bladder and cervix, and more rarely skin, regional lymph nodes, or lung.

The importance of the disease is given by its relatively high prevalence in women of reproductive age, its frequent association with infertility and with chronic pain, and its subsequent negative impact on the quality of life. Although many hypotheses have been postulated regarding the etiopathogenesis of endometriosis, its exact mechanisms remain unclear. Endometriosis is essentially a benign condition, but there are some common characteristics that suggest a connection to ovarian cancer, making the pathogenic pathways even more intriguing.

One element that supports the correlation between the two clinical entities is the fact that they share some epidemiological characteristics. These include the common risk factors, such as early onset of menstruation, short menstrual cycles, nulliparity, and late menopause, alongside the protective factors like oral contraceptive use, multiparity, tubal ligation, and hysterectomy [2]. Two primary mechanisms are hypothesized for this correlation: the direct malignant transformation of the endometriotic lesions or a combination of shared precursor mechanisms and risk factors, leading to distinct molecular pathways [3, 4].

The linkage between endometriosis and ovarian cancer was initially recognized under the term "endometriosis-associated ovarian carcinoma" (EAOC) [5] and subsequently referred to as "endometriosis-related ovarian neoplasm" (ERON) [6, 7] or "endometriosis-associated ovarian carcinoma" [8, 9], predominantly manifesting as endometrioid carcinoma, clear-cell carcinoma, seromucinous borderline tumors, Müllerian adenosarcoma, and endometrioid stromal sarcoma.

Notably, a majority of these tumors (70%) develop within the first decade following an endometriosis diagnosis, with 60% of cases exhibiting an intermediary stage of atypical endometriosis [9].

Furthermore, given the inherent invasive and metastatic abilities of endometriosis, its behavior closely resembles that of malignant conditions [10]. This profound connection has prompted investigations into potentially shared molecular pathways and the involvement of key molecules in their pathogenesis, thereby facilitating the assessment of endometriosis etiopathogenetic theories.

Regarding these molecular pathogenic pathways, a multitude of molecules have been studied in both endometriosis and EAOC. In this regard, estrogen is acknowledged as a promoter of ovarian cell proliferation, enhancing the mobility of malignant cells and inhibiting intercellular adhesion [11, 12]. The mediation by estrogen and progesterone receptors in the actions of steroid hormones on both endometriosis and endometrioid EAOC has been established, and recent studies have also correlated the expression of these receptors with clinical outcomes in ovarian cancer [12, 13]. Furthermore, p53 alterations also represent a significant molecular event in the transformation of endometriosis into carcinomas [14]. Similarly, Ki-67 expression, which is closely associated with cell proliferation, is employed to evaluate the growth of various neoplastic lesions, including both endometriosis and EAOC [15].

2. EAOC risk factors

Endometriosis is a condition relatively often associated with various types of neoplasms. EAOC occurs in 5–10% of endometriosis cases, and an intermediate stage of atypical endometriosis can be detected in 0.7–1.6% of cases [16]. A recent meta-analysis of 24 observational studies evaluated the link between endometriosis and ovarian cancer, revealing a calculated summary relative risk of 1.93 for ovarian cancer in women diagnosed with endometriosis compared to those without the condition [17].

In order to assess the individual risk for EAOC among endometriosis patients, Thomsen et al. have shown that in a group of women over the age of 45 years with endometriosis, factors, such as nulliparity, postmenopausal status, larger endometriomas (>9 cm), and either endogenous or exogenous hyperestrogenism, along with the presence of cysts containing solid components, were identified as risk indicators for EAOC [18].

Regarding the risk for a specific histological type of EAOC, a recent study has utilized genetic markers as proxies for epithelial ovarian cancer. The analysis revealed a significant correlation between these entities, with an odds ratio (OR) of 1.23. More detailed analysis, investigating for specific ovarian cancer histotypes possibly linked to endometriosis, showed an association of endometriosis with the risk of endometrioid carcinoma, clear-cell carcinoma, and low malignant potential tumors [19].

Some researchers have hypothesized the influence of the microenvironment, specifically the high iron concentration in the walls of endometriotic cysts in cases with prolonged evolution, through the persistence of oxidative stress induced by iron, resulting in subsequent DNA damage and numerous genetic mutations, such as PTEN (phosphatase and tensin homolog), ARID1 (AT-rich interactive domain-containing protein 1), PIK3CA (phosphatidylinositol-4,5-bisphosphate 3-kinase catalytic subunit alpha), and loss of heterozygosity [16].

Oncogenic mutations of the β-catenin phosphorylation site (catenin beta 1 (CTNNB1)) lead to the formation of a stable protein, detected both in endometriosis and in EAOC associated with endometriosis [16].

A significant role in the pathogenesis of endometriosis should be attributed to polygenic susceptibility, which implies a metabolic, endocrine, and immune association responsible for decreased immune surveillance, alongside pelvic inflammation [20–22].

Additionally, progressive accumulations of genetic alterations in tumor suppressor genes and oncogenes are likely responsible for the development of endometriosis and its possible association with the development of malignant conditions [23–29]. Premalignant lesions (atypical endometriosis) are characterized by multiple mutations in tumor suppressor genes, oncogenes, cell adhesion molecule (CAM), as well as loss of heterozygosity (LOH) and inflammatory immunomodulation [30].

3. Pathogeny/molecular mechanisms involved in the development of endometriosis and EAOC

Various endometriosis pathogenic pathways make this condition very similar to neoplastic processes. Among the widest spread and accepted pathogenetic theories in endometriosis are retrograde menstruation, immune dysregulation, coelomic metaplasia, hematogenous or lymphatic spread, endometrial stem cell recruitment theory, bone marrow-derived stem cells, alteration in epigenetic regulation, hormonal imbalance, and microRNAs (miRNAs). Besides these theories, the carcinogenetic pathways and external environmental factors are also believed to have a significant impact on endometriosis behavior and outcome [31, 32]. Although first proposed in the late nineteenth century, the most recently introduced hypothesis is the embryogenetic theory with Müllerian remnants' induction [32]. This is considered a type of metaplasia theory [31], stipulating that remnants of embryonic cells of Müllerian or Wolffian duct may transform into endometriotic lesions [31], by spreading the primordial endometrial cells towards the posterior pelvic floor during embryogenesis [32]. Most clinicians and theoreticians agree upon the menstrual reflux theory, which implies that endometrial cells are being expelled during menstruation, via the fallopian tubes, into the peritoneal cavity. Here, under yet unknown influences, these cells gain the capacity of adhesion to the peritoneal surface, invasion of the peritoneal lining, and further cellular survival and division. Their ectopic surviving capacity is provided by a mechanism of escaping the immune supervision of these newly formed implants. Furthermore, these implants have the capacity of neoangiogenesis, which promotes growth and development by providing nutrients and growth factors to the already-established implants.

Although a key role is attributed to the reflux of stem cells into the peritoneal cavity, the microenvironmental factors that stimulate stem cell functions and allow the development of endometriotic implants are very important as adjuvants to the mechanism of retrograde menstruation. Relatively recent data have demonstrated the existence of mesenchymal stem cells and endometrial progenitor cells in endometriosis and their potential evolution towards differentiation into nine cell lines, as follows: adipocytic, osteogenic, cardiomyocytic, respiratory epithelial, neurocytic, myocytic, endothelial, pancreatic, and hepatic [33]. Considering the widespread distribution of endometriosis in the human body, modern theories attempt to combine the effect of multiple factors contributing to its development, as multifactorial, multi-compartmental pathogenic phenomena, associated with epiphenomena, such as estrogen dependence [34], genetic susceptibility [35], and the possibility of direct spread through "transplantation" [34]. These processes add to the immune system's inability to neutralize ectopic endometrial cells [36–39], environmental factors, and the coexistence of congenital defects, such as hymenal atresia, for example. Last but not least, the most plausible pathogenic mechanism involves stem cells as the main factors responsible for the process of ectopic implantation via retrograde menstruation. The evasion of immune clearance, as the first step in the development of endometriotic lesions, is supported by various studies suggesting a modification of the immune system. Endometriosis may be associated with autoimmune diseases (systemic lupus erythematosus, rheumatoid arthritis, Sjögren's syndrome, autoimmune thyroiditis, and multiple sclerosis) or atopic diseases (allergies, asthma, and eczema) [40]. Considering that multiple autoantibodies can be identified in endometriosis [41], it may be considered that this autoimmune reactivity could be a consequence of chronic inflammation. In the last decade, studies have identified genetic, angiogenetic [42], endocrine, metabolic, and immunological anomalies, such that the pathogenesis of endometriosis is multifactorial, multi-compartmental, and associated with epiphenomena, many of which represent, in fact, consequences of the primary lesion.

Neoplastic transformation of some of these endometriotic implants has been a subject of research and debate. Nearly a century ago, John A. Sampson first identified ectopic endometrium-like tissue as a potential cause of ovarian carcinoma. He proposed that "metastatic or embolic endometriosis results from the menstrual dissemination of endometrial tissue into the venous circulation" [43]. This idea of retrograde menstruation leading to the implantation of endometrial cells in the peritoneal cavity, eventually transforming into ovarian cancer through atypical endometriosis, has since been widely studied. It seems that the ovarian microenvironment plays specific role in this malignant transformation [44], as it is an essential condition of such neoplasia. Even though endometriosis might have other locations, except the ovary, these sites are almost never the site of a malignant transformation [44, 45]. For example, the literature provides reports of only a few cases of carcinomas arising in rectovaginal endometriosis [46, 47].

Regarding the intermediate steps between endometriosis and EAOC, Kurman et al. [48] proposed the eutopic endometrium as the precursor site of origin of EAOC, endometriosis as the potential precursor lesion, and atypical endometriosis as the immediate precursor lesion. In the same context, Karnezis et al. consider endometriosis as the tissue of origin of EAOC, endometrial epithelial cells as the cells of origin, and endometrioid borderline tumors as the precursor lesion [49]. They also propose a classification of endometriosis as "high risk" and "low risk" depending on the presence of atypical endometriosis.

The molecular features of EAOC have been intensely studied in the last few years, and the results lead to different conclusions, depending on the type of EAOC. In this regard, endometriosis is considered a precursor to two completely different histological entities, endometriosis-associated ovarian clear-cell carcinoma (OCCC) and endometriosis-associated ovarian endometrioid carcinoma, without any recurrent genetic mutation that is unique to either of them [50].

3.1 Genetic mutations

Several genetic mutations have been identified as key drivers in the malignant transformation of endometriosis and the development of endometriosis-associated ovarian cancer (EAOC). Common mutations include those in p53, K-ras (Kirsten rat sarcoma virus), ARID1A, PIK3CA, and PPP2R1A (serine/threonine-protein phosphatase 2A regulatory subunit A). Although breast cancer (BRCA) mutations are prevalent in ovarian carcinomas, they are less frequently associated with EAOC [51].

Mutations in the ARID1A gene, which encodes the BAF250a (BRG-associated factor 250a) protein—a critical component of the switch/sucrose non-fermentable (SWI/SNF) adenosine triphosphate (ATP)-dependent chromatin remodeling complex—are found in nearly half of clear-cell and endometrioid carcinomas [52]. Loss of BAF250a in EAOC tissues is associated with increased expression of gamma H2A histone family member (γH2AX), a marker for DNA damage response, of the pro-apoptotic regulators, such as B-cell lymphoma 2-interacting mediator (BIM) and Bcl-2-associated X-protein (BAX), and decreased expression of the anti-apoptotic gene B-cell lymphoma 2 (Bcl-2). These findings suggest that chromatin remodeling and DNA damage response pathways may be involved in the early stages of precancerous lesions. ARID1A also shares downstream targets with p53, and its loss can lead to the dysregulation of p53-controlled genes [53].

In clear-cell EAOC, somatic mutations in the PIK3CA gene, which encodes a catalytic subunit of phosphatidylinositol-3 kinases (PI3K), often occur early and frequently coincide with the loss of ARID1A protein expression, potentially having synergistic effects [54]. Additional early markers in ARID1A-deficient carcinomas include the activation of RAC-alpha serine/threonine-protein kinase (AKT) through increased AKT serine/threonine kinase 1 (AKT1) expression and phosphorylation (phosphorylated AKT (pAKT)). Moreover, differential expression of components in the mammalian target of rapamycin (mTOR) pathway appears to link endometriosis with ovarian cancer development [53].

A less frequent mutation found in approximately 16–19% of EOAC and ovarian clear-cell carcinoma (OCCC) cases affects the oncogene PPP2R1A (serine/threonine-protein phosphatase 2A 65 kDa regulatory subunit A alpha isoform), which encodes a regulatory subunit of serine/threonine phosphatase 2 (PP2A), a negative regulator of cell growth [55].

Overall, the PI3K/protein kinase B (AKT)/mTOR pathway plays a critical role in cell cycle regulation, and mutations that alter gene regulation within this pathway contribute to the development and progression of ovarian cancer, as well as the transformation of healthy endometrial tissue into endometriosis and EAOC [56]. In contrast, the activity of the phosphatase and tensin homolog (PTEN), which counteracts the PI3K/AKT pathway, is diminished due to PTEN silencing in EAOC, thus reducing PTEN's inhibitory effect on cell growth and division [57].

Er et al. identified additional mutated genes in the Wnt pathway, the MAPK/ERK (mitogen-activated protein kinase/extracellular signal-regulated kinase 1/2) pathway, the Notch signaling pathway, cell cycle regulation, and the mismatch repair system through targeted next-generation sequencing [58]. Notably, the Notch signaling pathway is also disrupted in endometriosis and has been implicated in its pathogenesis [53].

3.2 Epigenetic mechanisms

Beyond genetic mutations, epigenetic mechanisms also play a crucial role in the malignant transformation of endometriosis into EAOC. For example, promoter hypermethylation can lead to the transcriptional inactivation of the MutL protein homolog 1 (MLH1) gene, which encodes a DNA mismatch repair (MMR) protein. This inactivation results in microsatellite instability and the accumulation of spontaneous mutations, thereby advancing the progression towards EAOC [59]. Additionally, other differentially methylated genes, such as Ras association domain family member 2 (RASSF2), which encodes the Kirsten rat sarcoma viral oncogene homolog (KRAS)- specific effector protein Ras association domain-containing protein 2, and Runt-related transcription factor 3 (RUNX3), which encodes the tumor-suppressing Runt-related transcription factor 3, have been identified as potential contributors to this malignant transformation [60].

3.3 The tumor microenvironment

The tumor microenvironment is crucial in shaping EAOCs, with estrogen concentration being a significant factor. High estrogen levels, whether from external sources like hormone replacement therapy or produced endogenously by the ovaries, promote the proliferation of endometriotic cells. Estrogen signaling in EAOC is complex and influenced by factors, such as nutritional status, oxidative stress, and surrounding cells, which in turn affect cellular metabolism, epithelial-to-mesenchymal transition (EMT), angiogenesis, and invasiveness [53].

microRNAs (miRNAs) are emerging as important posttranscriptional regulators of gene expression and potential biomarkers in endometriosis and EAOC. These small non-coding RNA (ncRNA) molecules can silence genes by binding to complementary sequences in messenger RNA (mRNA), leading to RNA degradation or translational repression. Dysregulation of miRNAs, such as those in the microRNA-200 (miR-200) and lethal-7 (let-7) families, has been observed in ovarian cancer and is involved in processes like the epithelial-to-mesenchymal transition and tumor progression [53]. Of note, microRNA-200b (miR-200b) also plays a role in the development of endometriosis, targeting zinc finger E-box-binding homeobox 1 (ZEB1), zinc finger E-box-binding homeobox 2 (ZEB2), and Kruppel-like factor 4 (KLF4), in order to regulate the stem cell phenotype, the proliferation, invasiveness, and the growth of invasive protrusions of endometriotic cells [61].

Szubert et al. found that the expression levels of microRNA-31-3p (miR-31-3p) and miR-200b were reduced in cancerous lesions compared to normal ovarian tissue and endometriosis tissue [62]. microRNA 31 (miR-31) activates hypoxia-inducible factor (HIF) under normoxic conditions by targeting the 3′ untranslated region (3′ UTR) of factor-inhibiting hypoxia-inducible factor (HIF), which leads to increased production of vascular endothelial growth factor (VEGF). VEGF overexpression is linked to both endometriosis and the progression to EAOC [53]. Furthermore, reduced levels of other microRNAs, including microRNA-17-5p (miR-17-5p), microRNA 20a (miR-20a), microRNA 222 (miR-222), and microRNA 125a (miR-125a), have been associated with angiogenesis in endometriosis by regulating factors, such as Runt-related transcription factor 1 (RUNX1), connective tissue growth factor (CTGF), thrombospondin-1 (TSP-1), and vascular endothelial growth factor-A (VEGF-A) [53].

Oxidative stress is another key factor in the malignant transformation of endometriosis to EAOC. microRNAs regulate oxidative stress by controlling the expression of reactive oxygen species (ROS)-related enzymes. Persistent oxidative stress in endometriotic cysts, possibly due to the release of free iron during menstruation, may contribute to their carcinogenic transformation [53].

Inflammation plays a significant role in EAOC carcinogenesis by creating a pro-tumorigenic environment that promotes DNA damage, tissue remodeling, immune suppression, and angiogenesis. Several inflammatory cytokines, complement factors, and inflammasome-related genes have been identified as contributors to the development of EAOC [53].

The tumor's ability to adapt to local nutrient availability through metabolic reprogramming is another emerging hallmark of cancer. Endometriotic cells often prefer aerobic glycolysis to generate energy, even in the presence of oxygen, which helps them survive in the extrauterine environment. Ovarian cancer cells exhibit metabolic heterogeneity and flexibility, allowing cancer cells to adapt to varying levels of glucose, lipids, and amino acids, thus contributing to their proliferation and survival [53].

It is considered that 2% of ovarian endometriotic lesions will undergo malignant transformation [63]. The exact etiopathology remains unclear, but both intrinsic factors within the endometrial tissue and microenvironmental factors are considered contributors to its survival in the peritoneum and potential malignant transformation [64]. For example, the increased frequency of chromosomal abnormalities in ovarian endometriosis, as opposed to extragonadal endometriosis, suggests that the ovarian stromal environment may play a role in initiating genetic alterations, possibly leading to invasive cancer [53].

In summary, the genetic profiles of benign ovaries and ovarian endometriosis differ significantly from those of EAOC and ovarian cancer [65].

The endometriosis-associated ovarian clear-cell carcinoma harbors mutations in ARID1A, PIK3CA, CTNNB1, and PTEN, while endometriosis-associated ovarian endometrioid carcinoma harbors mutations in PTEN, CTNNB1, KRAS, ARID1A, PPP2R1A, and PIK3CA [50].

Inactivating ARID1A mutations are the most common molecular genetic alterations reported in EAOC [66], resulting in loss of expression of the protein encoded by ARID1A (BAF250a). When expressed, this protein normally suppresses cellular proliferation through a p53-dependent transcription regulation of several tumor suppressors including CDKN1A (cyclin-dependent kinase inhibitor 1A) (encoding p21) and SMAD3 (mothers against decapentaplegic homolog 3) [67].

4. Pathological characteristics of ovarian endometriosis, atypical endometriosis, and EAOC

4.1 Endometriosis

On gross examination, endometriomas or ovarian endometriotic cysts present fibrotic walls, with smooth lining and characteristic dark brown content (chocolate cyst) [68].

If endometriosis has a polypoid aspect, it leads to the differential diagnosis of a neoplasm both on grossing and frozen sections [69]. Sometimes, the cyst can display red-brown or white plaques, with a gelatinous consistency [70, 71].

For the histopathological diagnosis of endometriosis, at least two of three criteria are needed: endometrial-type glands, lined by Müllerian-type epithelium, sometimes with degenerative atypia (enlarged faded nuclei) or metaplasia, included in an endometrial-type stroma. Sometimes, smooth muscle metaplasia, osseous metaplasia, decidual change, or myxoid aspects are found [72, 73]. Another rare and particular aspect is the presence of epithelial metaplastic changes or metaplasia in ovarian endometriosis, which should not be considered neoplastic features. A study conducted by Fukunaga on 315 cases of ovarian endometriosis found 162 cases with metaplastic changes, all of them being associated with atypical endometriosis or malignant ovarian epithelial tumor. Although no significant relationship was identified between the type of metaplasia in endometriosis and the type of carcinoma, mucinous metaplasia was correlated with cases of Müllerian mucinous borderline tumors, and thus there could be an association between this type of metaplasia and hyperplasia encountered in ovarian endometriosis and Müllerian mucinous borderline ovarian tumors [74].

Moreover, there are cases when the histopathological diagnosis is made only on the presence of endometrial stroma (stromal endometriosis) or indirectly, due to the chronic hemorrhage, with foamy or hemosiderin-laden macrophages. Rarely, Liesegang rings, defined as eosinophilic noncellular rings embedded in necrotic tissue or necrotic pseudoxanthomatous nodules, with central necrosis bounded by histiocytes and an outer fibrous tissue are encountered [72]. Somewhat similar morphological aspects as mentioned above, suggestive of endometriosis, define the so-called "burnt out endometriosis."

4.2 Atypical endometriosis

Atypical endometriosis was reported in 1.74.4% of endometriotic ovarian cysts, being considered as the precursor lesion for EAOC, mainly endometrioid or clear-cell type. Atypical endometriotic lesions were found in association with these tumors in 25% of cases, presenting the same genomic alterations as EAOC [75]. Histopathological landscape is characterized by crowded endometrial-type glands, with complex architecture, lined by atypical epithelial cells as those observed in atypical endometrial hyperplasia (AEH) [75–77].

Atypical endometriosis (AE) has been historically described as having histological characteristics that are intermediary between benign and malignant states, including enlarged atypical hyperchromatic nuclei, an elevated nuclear-to-cytoplasm ratio, and cellular overcrowding, sometimes with hobnail features [75–79]. This type of lesion has been found to sometimes coexist with endometriosis and more frequently with EAOC, and it involves changes in the epithelial lining of endometriotic cysts marked by varying levels of cellular stratification, disorganization, inflammation, and cytological atypia [8, 77].

AE has been proposed as a precancerous lesion, as studies have shown that it can be considered as a transitional state between endometriosis and EAOC. In this regard, Ogawa et al. have reevaluated microscopic slides from 127 patients with primary ovarian carcinoma and concluded that 37 patients also had endometriosis, from which 29 cases had atypical endometriosis. The study reported the transition from typical endometriosis to AE in 22 cases, and the transition from AE to carcinoma in 23 cases, suggesting an AE could be considered a precancerous lesion, even though it is not encountered in all cases [80].

In order to further refine the risk of EAOC in the AE cases, Stamp et al. suggested that BAF250a expression may be a biomarker of cancer risk in patients diagnosed with atypical endometriosis. In their study, which included 35 cases of EAOC and 8 cases of non-cancerous AE, the immunohistochemical (IHC) expression of BAF250a was lost in most of the cases of AE associated with EAOC, but not in non-cancerous AE [81].

4.3 Endometriosis-associated ovarian cancers

The main epithelial ovarian cancer histotypes are classified as types I and II, according to the dualistic pathogenic model proposed by Kurman et al. [48]. The first category comprises the so-called endometriosis-associated tumors and it includes the endometrioid, clear-cell, and seromucinous carcinomas. Type II tumors are mainly composed of high-grade serous carcinomas, which represent almost the majority (70%) of ovarian carcinomas [48]. Among the EAOC, the seromucinous histotype is rare, while the most frequent histotypes associated with endometriosis are the endometrioid ovarian carcinomas and the clear-cell ovarian carcinomas. One essential difference between the two categories resides in their pathogenic models and their subsequent prognosis.

It is now considered that most high-grade serous carcinomas originate from undetectable atypical lesions within the fallopian tubes [82], with subsequent exfoliation and implantation on the ovaries, peritoneum, omentum and on abdominopelvic organs, resulting in the development of late-stage cancers from inception. In contrast, most of the type I tumors originate from ovarian endometriotic cysts that are easily detected, and they are confined to the ovary for a variable period of time, making therapeutic approaches more efficient and improving the prognosis [48].

To conclude, EAOC typically manifests as endometrioid and clear-cell carcinomas, and less frequently by seromucinous borderline tumors, squamous cell carcinoma, carcinosarcoma, adenosarcoma, or endometrial stromal sarcoma.

4.3.1 Endometrioid carcinomas

Endometrioid carcinomas represent 25% of ovarian carcinomas [83]. Regardless of the disease stage or response to platinum-based therapies, the prognosis is favorable. It has been found that patients diagnosed with endometrioid ovarian carcinoma often have a clinical history and microscopic foci of endometriosis (10–20%) [84]. Squamous differentiation, a pathognomonic element for ovarian endometrioid tumors, is found in about half of the cases associated with endometriosis. Morphologically, ovarian endometrioid carcinomas exhibit an endometrioid-like epithelium, similar to uterine endometrioid carcinomas, characterized by stratified columnar, non-mucinous, with a villoglandular pattern. Most tumor glands present luminal margins, oriented back-to-back, separated by an abundant fibrocellular stroma. Ovarian endometrioid carcinoma exhibits the following architectural patterns: papillary, cribriform, glandular, microglandular, spindle cell, secretory, ciliated cell, sertoliform, and sex cord-like [85]. Based on nuclear grade and the percentage of solid area, ovarian endometrioid carcinomas are classified as: well, moderately, or poorly differentiated. If the well-differentiated type presents a villoglandular architecture, the moderately and poorly differentiated types are most frequently solid, glandular, or microglandular. Cellular atypia and mitotic figures are rarely encountered in poorly differentiated carcinomas, while high-grade tumors exhibit marked nuclear pleomorphism, associated with an increased mitotic index. In the situation of an undifferentiated pattern of ovarian carcinoma, the following criteria favor a diagnosis of endometrioid carcinoma: (i) metaplastic structural elements, such as squamous, morular, mucinous, or "hobnail," (ii) cellular phenotype (eosinophilic cells or secretory changes), (iii) foci of endometriosis, and (iv) fibrous stroma [85].

4.3.2 Clear-cell carcinomas

Clear-cell carcinomas represent approximately 5% of ovarian carcinomas [83]. The characteristic feature of these tumors is that, regardless of the grading type used, they have an unfavorable progression, often recur compared to other histological types, and have a reduced response rate to chemotherapy (CHT) [84]. Thus, compared to other tumor types, although they are included in the category of type I tumors, these are high-grade, with a reserved prognosis. The latest trends according to the specialized literature suggest including ovarian clear-cell carcinomas in the category of type II tumors. The etiopathogenesis of this category is closely related to endometriosis, similar to ovarian endometrioid tumors. Morphologically, ovarian clear-cell carcinomas have three essential features to be followed: (i) cytoplasmic changes, (ii) nuclear appearance, and (iii) architectural pattern. Due to the "clear" appearance of the cellular cytoplasm (resulting from the accumulation of glycogen) or the eosinophilic appearance (oxyphil cells), clear-cell carcinomas are easily recognized. It should be noted that, for histopathologists, just the clear cytoplasmic appearance is not sufficient for diagnosis, as this appearance can occur not only as a result of glycogen accumulation but also of lipids or as a result of cellular injury with a hydropic-vacuolar cytoplasmic appearance. The particular nuclear appearance gives the cell a "target" shape, "hobnail," characterized by hyperchromatic nuclei that protrude into the glandular lumen. The most frequently encountered architectural phenotypes in clear-cell carcinomas are: tubulocystic/cystic (dilated cystic glands lined by flattened epithelium), papillary (small round papillary axes lined by epithelium with a maximum of two layers of polygonal or cuboidal cells), and the solid pattern, with mucin-containing cytoplasm (rarely described). Characteristically, all described patterns are located in a hyalinized, eosinophilic, fibroblastic, myxoid, rarely colloid stroma. The increased mitotic index, stratification, and cellular detachment are not characteristic of ovarian clear-cell carcinomas [86]. Occasionally, cellular features such as "signet ring" cells can be identified [86]. Additionally, morphological features, such as open tumor rings, hyaline globules, and targetoid bodies, have been described [86].

4.3.3 Borderline seromucinous tumors

Borderline seromucinous tumors were historically designated as borderline Müllerian mucinous or borderline endocervical-type or mixed epithelial papillary borderline tumor of Müllerian type or atypical proliferative tumors, and these terms are not currently being used. They constitute a small proportion of ovarian mucinous borderline tumors (10–15%) [7, 8] and are associated, in about one-third to half of cases, with endometriosis [8, 45]. Cytologically, these tumors exhibit a stratified epithelium containing a combination of endocervical-type mucosecretory cells, ciliated cells, and occasional acidophilic cells with abundant cytoplasm [7, 45], alongside a wide range of possible differentiations (endometrioid, serous, clear cell, and squamous) [8], most commonly presenting a low degree of atypia [8]. These tumors are often bilateral [8], are associated with stromal microinvasion [8] and although most of them are detected at an early stage, some may present peritoneal implants, as in the case of borderline serous tumors [7], and even lymph node involvement [45].

In terms of potential pathogenic mechanisms, the hypothesis of a mucinous metaplasia within endometriosis followed by progression to a cystadenoma and borderline tumor has been proposed [45].

This type of tumor shares the genetic profile of endometrioid tumor [8] and has a favorable prognosis [7]. Rarely, the malignant character associated with the borderline nature is observed, suggestive of tumor progression and having negative implications for the prognosis [8].

Due to the low degree of diagnostic concordance among gynecological pathologists and the immunohistochemical pattern of low-grade endometrioid or serous tumors, this diagnostic category remains controversial, suggesting its classification as a subtype of another type of ovarian tumor [8].

4.3.4 Carcinosarcoma

Carcinosarcoma, also known as malignant mixed Müllerian tumor or malignant mixed mesodermal tumor, morphologically represents a combination of malignant epithelial components, often high-grade (typically serous or endometrioid, and rarely undifferentiated) and mesenchymal components, either homologous or heterologous (such as osteosarcoma, rhabdomyosarcoma, chondrosarcoma, angiosarcoma, or liposarcoma) [7, 45]. These tumors frequently associate with serous tubal intraepithelial carcinoma [8] and, in about 50% of cases, with endometriosis [7].

Patients are most commonly over 50 years old, and the diagnosis is typically made in advanced stages [7]. Generally, the tumors are predominantly solid, large, with areas of cystic degeneration [45], and often exhibit extraovarian extension as they progress [7]. According to recent studies on the immunohistochemical and molecular profile, carcinosarcomas are included in the category of carcinomas that undergo stromal differentiation [8].

4.3.5 Adenosarcoma

Adenosarcoma is a neoplasm characterized by the association of a benign epithelial component with a malignant mesenchymal component, typically low-grade [7]. This biphasic tumor typically exhibits a morphology where glands are seen associated with periglandular stromal hypercellularity, displaying a papillary or polypoid appearance, with mild-to-moderate cytologic atypia, analogous to a phyllodes tumor [7]. Within this tumor, elements of sex cord development and the development of a high-grade sarcomatous component, typically with rhabdomyosarcomatous differentiation, can be associated [8, 45].

From a clinical progression standpoint, about 50% of patients exhibit extraovarian tumor extension [7]. Due to easy peritoneal dissemination, the possibility of tumor rupture, and overdevelopment of high-grade stroma, this type of tumor presents a reserved prognosis, particularly in younger patients [7, 8, 45].

Recent data from molecular studies have demonstrated that these tumors belong to the category of mesenchymal neoplasms [8].

4.3.6 Endometrioid stromal sarcoma

Morphologically, endometrioid stromal sarcoma is a frequently bilateral ovarian tumor that exhibits a morphology similar to that of endometrial stroma [7], with high-grade cytologic atypia associated with marked mitotic activity [45]. It has been observed that about 50% of patients with this tumor have it in the context of endometriosis [7].

Microscopically, endometrioid stromal sarcoma associated with endometriosis consists of large spindle cells with an increased nuclear to cytoplasm ratio, associated with spiral-like arterioles, and is more often low-grade than high-grade [7, 45].

In the literature, there is a reported possibility of association between ovarian endometrioid stromal sarcoma and synchronous or preexisting endometrial sarcoma, sharing a common cytogenetic profile [7, 8].

Ovarian endometrioid stromal sarcoma is often diagnosed at advanced stages and has a reserved prognosis [45].

4.3.7 Squamous cell carcinoma

Rarely, primary ovarian squamous cell carcinoma, possibly associated with squamous metaplasia, can occur in a context of endometriosis [7].

Although cases of non-invasive squamous neoplasia with a flat or papillary appearance within ovarian cysts, associated with cervical intraepithelial neoplasia, have been described, the suspicion of the role of human papillomavirus (HPV) has been ruled out in the etiopathogenesis of ovarian involvement due to HPV negativity at the ovarian level [7].

5. Evaluation of a suspicious endometriotic lesion

5.1 Clinical evaluation

Given that 90% of ovarian masses in premenopausal women and 60% of those in postmenopausal women prove to be benign [87], assessing the neoplastic risk is crucial in guiding diagnostic and therapeutic techniques. The suspicion of malignant transformation is difficult to determine before surgical exploration, as ovarian carcinoma is known as a "silent killer," typically diagnosed in advanced stages. However, some symptoms and clinical signs can raise an alarm several months before diagnosis, even from the early stages [88], indicating the necessity for additional preoperative investigations that can facilitate an optimal diagnostic and therapeutic approach. Before initiating surgical treatment, obtaining a complete medical history, including significant familial and genetic risk assessments, is mandatory.

Physical examination may reveal an abdominopelvic mass with characteristics suggestive of tumor transformation: solid, firm, nodular, fixed to surrounding anatomical structures. It should be noted that a very large tumor mass often proves to be a benign or borderline tumor. Rectovaginal examination is important in planning surgical intervention, as if infiltration of the rectovaginal septum is observed, a low anterior resection (of the rectosigmoid) may be necessary.

If the clinical examination reveals ascitic fluid associated with a pelvic mass, an ovarian neoplasm diagnosis should be considered, until proven otherwise. Evidently, if there is a suspicion of neoplasia, pulmonary auscultation is mandatory, which might identify pleurisy, as well as examination of the superficial lymph node groups.

5.2 Laboratory findings

Facing an endometriotic lesion with atypical appearance, a comprehensive evaluation is recommended, including a complete blood count. This is necessary before any surgical intervention and can provide additional clues, considering that 20–25% of patients with ovarian neoplasia also exhibit thrombocytosis (>400x10^9/L) [89]. Hyponatremia is also commonly identified, generally ranging between 125 and 135 mEq/L (milliequivalents per liter).

Among the tumor markers used to classify patients into risk groups are cancer antigen 125 (CA125) and human epididymis protein 4 (HE4). Additionally, two algorithms for calculating neoplastic risk, the "risk of ovarian malignancy algorithm" (ROMA) and the "risk malignancy index" (RMI), are utilized. The CA125 value is higher than the cutoff value of 35 U/mL in over 90% of cases of non-mucinous ovarian carcinoma, but interpretation must be cautious, as only 50% of stage I carcinomas exhibit this characteristic [90]. The marker also has low specificity, with elevated values also found in endometriosis, as well as in patients with benign gynecological pathology or in physiological conditions, such as menstruation, pregnancy, pelvic inflammatory disease, and also in abdominal diseases, especially liver or pancreatic conditions.

HE4 has a sensitivity of 72.9% and a specificity of 95% in differentiating benign from malignant ovarian tumors, both values being higher than those of CA125 [91]. The ROMA score takes into account the values of both markers, along with the patient's menopausal status, providing a sensitivity of 88.7% and a specificity of 74.7% [92]. As for the RMI, it additionally utilizes the ultrasonic features of the ovarian tumor, which enhances both the sensitivity and specificity of the evaluation.

5.3 Imaging techniques

To differentiate benign from malignant ovarian tumors, the most commonly used imaging technique is pelvic ultrasound. When employing this method, the International Ovarian Tumor Analysis (IOTA) 2018 score is used, which considers various ultrasonographic aspects of ovarian neoplasia. Characteristics suggestive of benignity include the presence of a unilocular cyst, solid components with a maximum diameter of 7 mm, acoustic shadows, a multilocular cyst with a smooth surface and maximum diameter of 100 mm, and the absence of blood flow. Indicators of malignancy include the presence of an irregular solid tumor, ascitic fluid, at least four papillary structures, an irregular multilocular solid tumor with a maximum diameter of 100 mm, and pronounced blood flow [93].

Ultrasound examination is less significant in advanced disease, as it is more difficult to interpret and cannot specify all the details necessary for staging. In such cases, CT scanning is preferred, which also allows for the assessment of hepatic, retroperitoneal, omental, or lymph node involvement and can identify the extension of the tumor to other locations. CT is not useful in differentiating benign from malignant ovarian tumor masses and is generally used to plan surgical intervention when there is a high suspicion of ovarian carcinoma. Other complementary imaging explorations include MRI and PET. Chest radiography is essential to detect pleural effusion or, less commonly, pulmonary metastases.

6. Prevention techniques

Identification of those endometriomas that contain foci of AE would allow preventive measures to be taken in a useful manner. This could lead to either a timely surgery that would prevent the progression towards invasive carcinoma or even conservative treatment if the malignancy is detected in early stages, considerably reducing the morbidity, the mortality, and the treatment costs.

Such measures currently include:

- early detection of EAOC;
- risk-reducing medical treatment;
- risk-reducing surgical treatment.

6.1 Early detection of EAOC

Early detection and treatment of endometriosis-associated ovarian cancer (EAOC), which primarily includes endometrioid and clear-cell ovarian carcinomas, significantly impact long-term outcomes for patients. It plays a crucial role in improving long-term outcomes for patients by increasing survival rates, reducing recurrence, enhancing quality of life, and expanding treatment options. Integrating effective screening and monitoring strategies into clinical practice can help achieve these benefits, ultimately leading to better patient outcomes.

Detecting EAOC at an early stage (I or II) significantly improves overall survival rates. Early-stage cancers are generally confined to the ovary or the pelvis, allowing for complete surgical removal, which is the cornerstone of treatment. Patients diagnosed at these stages typically have a much higher 5-year survival rate compared to those diagnosed at advanced stages (III or IV), where survival rates drop significantly.

When EAOC is detected early, the likelihood of achieving optimal cytoreduction (removal of all visible tumor tissue) is much higher. Complete surgical resection is a critical factor in improving survival, as it reduces tumor burden and enhances the effectiveness of adjuvant therapies like chemotherapy or targeted therapies. In contrast, advanced-stage disease often involves widespread metastasis, making complete surgical removal more challenging and reducing the chances of achieving optimal outcomes.

Also, early detection of EAOC can lead to a greater responsiveness to standard platinum-based chemotherapy, which is less effective in advanced, chemoresistant tumors, particularly clear-cell ovarian carcinomas. Early-stage tumors are generally smaller, less aggressive, and more likely to be effectively treated with standard chemotherapy regimens, which can help prevent recurrence and prolong progression-free survival. Early detection can reduce the need for aggressive, multi-modal treatments often required for advanced-stage EAOC. For early-stage disease, less extensive surgery, lower doses of chemotherapy, or the use of targeted therapies may suffice, minimizing the treatment-related toxicity and improving the quality of life for patients.

For younger patients diagnosed with early-stage EAOC who wish to preserve fertility, early detection allows for more conservative surgical options, such as unilateral salpingo-oophorectomy (removal of one ovary and fallopian tube) or cystectomy (removal of the cyst only). These approaches may maintain reproductive potential while still effectively treating the cancer, provided the disease is adequately staged and monitored.

Patients diagnosed with early-stage EAOC also have a lower risk of cancer recurrence compared to those diagnosed at a later stage. Early detection allows for complete resection of the tumor and a more effective initial treatment, reducing the likelihood of residual disease that could lead to recurrence. Lower recurrence rates are associated with better long-term survival and quality of life.

The early detection of EAOC could be obtained by a trained ultrasonographist, as this technique allows complete characterization of the location and extent of endometriotic lesions [94]. Supplementary MRI, when available, is useful in detecting all locations of endometriosis, especially when ultrasonography has limitations (for example, regarding lesions located above the rectosigmoid junction) [94].

In this context, several researchers have raised awareness towards the elements of suspicion, pointing out the signs and symptoms that might suggest malignant transformation of an endometriotic cyst. For example, Nezhat et al. point out that an increase of endometrioma size, changing of ultrasonographic characteristics, and mural node formation constitute ominous signs that require surgical excision [95]. Suspicion is also raised when the patient develops symptoms such as dysmenorrhea and dyspareunia or is facing a relapse or worsening pelvic pain symptoms [96]. Supplementary, advancing age (over 45 years) and the size of endometriomas (over 8 cm) were found to be independent predictors of development of ovarian cancer among women with ovarian endometrioma [50]. It is generally believed that when gynecologists or radiologists with specialized oncological experience evaluate all suspicious endometriomas, the effectiveness of imaging techniques in identifying cysts that need surgical removal can be significantly improved. [50].

In a recent article, Younis et al. postulate that the overall lifetime risk of a woman with endometriosis to develop EAOC remains minimal [97]. They emphasize the importance of imagistic differentiation between benign, "homogenous cystic 'ground glass'"-appearing endometrioma and EAOC. They consider that suspicious ultrasound findings, such as large, vascularized, papillary, unilateral cysts (>9 cm) with solid intracystic projections, should be further characterized by MRI [97, 98]. In this regard, the non-invasive transvaginal ultrasound is considered a new and promising technique in early diagnosis of malignant transformed endometriosis, being able to accurately evaluate ovarian masses, the method being doubled by MRI in uncertain cases [99].

6.2 Risk-reducing medical treatment

It is already established that prolonged oral contraceptive use is associated with a major reduction in the risk of developing an endometrioma, as this medication inhibits ovulation. It can be concluded that oral contraceptives and progestogens should theoretically reduce the risk of EAOC in women with a history of endometriosis, even in those without current endometriomas [50]. It is well known that the development of endometrioid ovarian cancer is primarily driven by a hormonal environment with high levels of estrogen and low levels of progesterone. Additionally, high intracystic levels of heme and free iron lead to a state of persistent oxidative stress, which may lead to stress-resistant types like clear-cell ovarian carcinoma. In this context, Kim et al. propose that the long-term use of oral contraceptives and progestogens in women with existing endometriomas may reduce the risk of mainly receptor-positive endometrioid ovarian cancer to a greater extent than with respect to the risk of mainly receptor-negative clear-cell ovarian carcinoma [100]. Overall, the long-term use of oral contraceptives might contribute to the prevention of EAOC by limiting disease progression without detrimental effects on the reproductive potential [101].

6.3 Risk-reducing surgical treatment

Regardless of the imagistic aspect and suspicion, some clinicians suggest surgery as a method of risk reduction. Even though in younger women diagnosed with endometrioma, surgery has specific individual indications and limits, in perimenopausal women removal of ovaries with endometriotic cysts may be taken into consideration. Until now, no robust studies have provided information regarding the effect of surveillance compared with that of surgery (unilateral salpingo-oophorectomy or cystectomy/partial ovarian excision) on mortality from EAOC in patients with endometriosis/endometriomas [50].

Specialists suggest that surgery should be considered for endometriomas with a prolonged evolution, especially if they are not being hormonally treated (either with oral contraceptives or with progestogens), and also in the case of de novo detection of an endometrioma during medical treatment, as the risk of malignancy appears here to have substantially increased [102, 103]. Moreover, according to Haraguchi et al., recurrent endometriomas are at especially augmented risk of malignant transformation, as all EAOCs in their series developed in patients who experienced a cyst recurrence [104]. In most women with a history of endometriosis but without ultrasonographic evidence of endometriomas, surveillance rather than risk-reducing salpingo-oophorectomy seems advisable.

6.4 Clinical applicability of identified risk factors

Identified risk factors for EAOC can be utilized in clinical practice to enhance screening, early detection, and prevention strategies.

Identifying high-risk individuals, such as personal history of endometriosis or family history of ovarian or endometrial cancer, could lead to a more personalized approach in order to provide them specific screening tools. Clinicians should consider more frequent monitoring and evaluation for ovarian cancer in women with a known history of endometriosis, particularly those with long-standing or severe endometriosis, including regular pelvic examinations, transvaginal ultrasounds, and potentially advanced imaging techniques like MRI, if warranted. Regular monitoring of serum biomarkers, such as CA125 and human epididymis protein 4 (HE4) in high-risk women, could help detect early signs of malignancy, although these markers have limitations in sensitivity and specificity. Combining biomarker analysis with imaging techniques may improve early detection rates.

Additionally, women with a family history of ovarian, endometrial, or breast cancer may be at increased risk, especially if there is a familial link to conditions like Lynch syndrome or BRCA mutations. Genetic counseling and testing can be offered to these patients to identify hereditary cancer syndromes and guide risk-reducing strategies, such as increased surveillance, chemoprevention, or risk-reducing surgeries.

For patients with endometriosis, molecular profiling of endometriotic lesions, if excised, may help identify mutations (e.g., ARID1A, PTEN) or hormonal profiles that are associated with higher malignancy risk. Women with these profiles may benefit from closer surveillance.

Clinicians could also implement some risk-reducing interventions, such as hormonal therapy or tailored surgical approaches. Long-term use of hormonal therapies, such as oral contraceptives or progestins, may reduce the risk of endometrioid ovarian cancer in women with endometriosis. Hormonal therapy can create a progesterone-dominant environment, which has been associated with a lower risk of malignant transformation of endometriotic lesions. For women with endometriosis who are considered at high risk for EAOC (e.g., due to family history or genetic mutations), risk-reducing surgeries, such as prophylactic oophorectomy (removal of the ovaries) or hysterectomy, may be discussed. Surgical removal of visible endometriotic lesions during laparoscopy can also reduce the risk of malignancy, especially for lesions that are atypical or recurrent.

Last but not least, patients could benefit from lifestyle modifications, education, and awareness. Encouraging lifestyle changes, such as maintaining a healthy weight, avoiding smoking, and managing stress, can be important preventive measures. While the direct impact of these factors on EAOC is less clear, a healthy lifestyle is generally protective against many forms of cancer. Educating patients with endometriosis about their potentially increased risk of ovarian cancer, particularly if they have additional risk factors, can empower them to participate actively in surveillance and prevention strategies. Patients should be informed of symptoms that could suggest malignant transformation, such as pelvic pain, bloating, or changes in menstrual patterns, and seek medical evaluation promptly.

Additionally, encouraging eligible high-risk women to participate in clinical trials aimed at identifying new screening tools, biomarkers, and preventive strategies could contribute to advancing the field and improving outcomes for EAOC.

7. Treatment

The traditional therapeutic approach included debulking surgery followed by adjuvant chemotherapy, with salvage chemotherapy as an option if the initial treatment failed or if there was a recurrence. Nevertheless, due to the recent progress in deciphering the intrinsic mechanisms of endometriosis and of EAOC, the treatment approach for EAOC has also evolved. The molecular and pathological characteristics of EAOC significantly influence treatment strategies and patient outcomes.

According to the current guidelines, chemotherapeutic option for ovarian drugs cancer commonly used in the treatment of ovarian cancer, including in the EAOC, includes platinum-based drugs, such as cisplatin and carboplatin, as well as taxanes, such as paclitaxel [105, 106].

However, in the advanced stages (FIGO (The International Federation of Gynecology and Obstetrics) stage III or IV) or recurrent cases, a declining effectiveness of chemotherapy was noted, leading to a poor prognosis. Consequently, there has been a shift towards enhancing the efficacy of first-line treatment. This involves prioritizing aggressive surgical cytoreduction to improve the quality of surgery and adopting newer chemotherapy agents, often combined with targeted therapy or immunotherapy, to enhance treatment outcomes. Also, hyperthermic intraperitoneal chemotherapy (HIPEC) with perfusion of intraperitoneal chemotherapy during the surgical intervention was introduced in the therapeutic arsenal.

Taking into account the strong hormone dependence of endometriosis and EAOC, hormonotherapy is currently used as another adjuvant systemic treatment option [105, 107]. For example, elevated levels of progesterone receptor (PR) in endometrioid ovarian carcinoma have been linked to a better prognosis and thus could be potential targets for tumors. In this context, high PR expression is generally associated with a more favorable prognosis and may guide the use of hormone-based therapies, such as progestins or anti-estrogen agents (e.g., tamoxifen).

Conversely, the loss of estrogen receptor alpha or the high expression of estrogen receptor beta and gamma have been associated with reduced overall survival in ovarian cancer [108, 109]. In this context, several recent studies have evaluated the therapeutic potential of endocrine agents, such as letrozole, tamoxifen, aromatase inhibitors, and fulvestrant, in ovarian cancer, as reviewed by Langdon et al. [110]. Supplementary, estradiol-triazole analogs were developed, with the scope of targeting proteins involved in the epidermal growth factor receptor/mitogen-activated protein kinase (EGFR/MAPK) pathway in ovarian cancer [111].

Another innovative strategy involves incorporating the anti-angiogenic medication bevacizumab, a monoclonal antibody that targets vascular endothelial growth factor (VEGF)-A, into first-line treatment alongside chemotherapy. Additionally, bevacizumab can be utilized as monotherapy for individuals with newly diagnosed advanced ovarian cancer and platinum-resistant recurrent cases. Moreover, clear-cell ovarian carcinoma often overexpresses VEGF and anti-angiogenic agents, such as bevacizumab, can be particularly effective for these tumors.

Moreover, oral VEGF receptor tyrosine kinase inhibitors like pazopanib and nintedanib have been employed for maintenance therapy in platinum-sensitive recurrent ovarian cancer, offering notable benefits [112].

The tumor microenvironment, including immune cell infiltration, can affect treatment responses. Tumors with high immune cell infiltration may be more responsive to immunotherapy, while those with a suppressed immune microenvironment might require combination treatments to enhance the immune response.

In addition to that, the advancement and utilization of anticancer immunotherapies, involving immune checkpoint inhibitors like anti-cytotoxic T-lymphocyte-associated protein 4 (CTLA-4) and anti-programmed cell death protein 1 (PD-1)/programmed death-ligand 1 (PD-L1) antibodies, have resulted in notable enhancements in the management of diverse cancers. These therapies are particularly effective in combating the evasion of immune-mediated detection and elimination of malignant cells [112].

Regarding the genetic mutations and alterations with potential therapeutic targeting, it has been shown that EAOCs frequently exhibit mutations in genes, such as ARID1A and PTEN, which are implicated in chromatin remodeling and cell growth regulation, respectively. These mutations can help identify tumors that might respond to targeted therapies, like PI3K/AKT/mTOR inhibitors.

Also, some EAOCs may show deficiencies in mismatch repair proteins, leading to microsatellite instability (MSI). These tumors are often more responsive to immune checkpoint inhibitors (e.g., pembrolizumab), making immunotherapy a viable treatment option.

Insights into molecular pathways of EAOCs could also lead a way towards personalized therapy. As clear-cell ovarian carcinoma often shows activation of the PI3K/AKT/mTOR pathway, it could be a potential candidate for mTOR inhibitors (e.g., everolimus) or PI3K inhibitors.

Further detailed analysis could provide insights regarding biomarkers for personalized treatment. The presence of specific biomarkers, such as hormone receptors, MSI status, and actionable mutations (e.g., BRCA, ARID1A), helps to stratify patients for personalized treatment approaches, potentially improving outcomes by tailoring therapies to the tumor's unique molecular profile.

8. Prognosis

Taking into consideration the particularities of EAOC, such as the high prevalence of endometrioid or clear-cell ovarian cancer (CCOC) histotypes, it is generally considered that it has a better prognosis than other types of ovarian cancer, with the exception of advanced stages of clear-cell ovarian cancer, which has an earlier recurrence rate and a lower overall survival rate [113]. In any case, EAOC is usually detected sooner than non-EAOC, which also contributes to the better management and prognosis of this neoplasia, but it is unclear whether the association with endometriosis actually contributes to this better prognosis, compared to endometrial cancer (EC) and CCOC, which are not associated with endometriosis [113]. Similar conclusions were reached by Li et al. [114], who concluded that in patients with EAOCs, a significantly longer overall survival was recorded compared to non-EAOC patients, probably because the association with endometriosis leads to a higher prevalence of early-stage and low-grade tumors, and thus a much better survival rate than non-EAOC. These survival analysis findings showed that stage at diagnosis seems to be more important to prognosis than association with endometriosis alone [114]. Ultimately, the molecular and pathological characteristics of EAOC significantly influence treatment strategies and outcomes. By understanding these characteristics, clinicians can better tailor therapies to individual patients, potentially improving response rates and survival outcomes.

In conclusion, endometriosis-associated ovarian cancer (EAOC), encompassing primarily endometrioid and clear-cell ovarian carcinomas, represents a distinct subset of ovarian malignancies with unique molecular and pathological characteristics that directly influence patient management and outcomes. Early detection remains pivotal, as it markedly improves survival rates, enhances responsiveness to standard treatments, and allows for more conservative approaches, including fertility preservation in younger patients. Understanding the role of hormonal environments, genetic mutations, and the molecular pathways driving the transformation from endometriosis to EAOC has led to more personalized treatment strategies and improved patient care.

However, significant gaps in knowledge persist. Future research should focus on developing reliable, non-invasive biomarkers and advanced imaging techniques for early detection, particularly in high-risk women. Additionally, a deeper understanding of the molecular mechanisms underlying the progression of endometriosis to malignancy is crucial to identifying new therapeutic targets. Research should also explore the role of the tumor microenvironment and the immune system's involvement in EAOC progression to optimize the use of immunotherapies and targeted treatments. Addressing these unresolved questions will be key to advancing the field, improving early detection, and ultimately providing better outcomes for patients with EAOC.

Author details

Ioana Pavaleanu*, Teodora Ana Balan, Tiberiu Nicolae Poparlan, Ana Maria Haliciu, Tudor Andrei Butureanu, Ana Maria Apetrei, Razvan Socolov, Andreea Ioana Pruteanu and Raluca Anca Balan
Gr. T. Popa University of Medicine and Pharmacy, Iași, Romania

*Address all correspondence to: ioana_pavaleanu@yahoo.com

References

[1] Audebert A, Petousis S, Margioula-Siarkou C, Ravanos K, Prapas N, Prapas Y. Anatomic distribution of endometriosis: A reappraisal based on series of 1101 patients. European Journal of Obstetrics, Gynecology, and Reproductive Biology. 2018;**230**:36-40

[2] Van Gorp T, Amant F, Neven P, et al. Endometriosis and the development of malignant tumours of the pelvis. A review of literature. Best Practice & Research. Clinical Obstetrics & Gynaecology. 2004;**18**:349-371

[3] Hanahan D, Weinberg RA. The hallmarks of cancer. Cell. 2000;**100**(1):57-70

[4] Hanahan D, Weinberg RA. The hallmarks of cancer: The next generation. Cell. 2011;**144**(5):646-674

[5] Scott R. Malignant change in endometriosis. Obstetrics and Gynecology. 1953;**2**:293-299

[6] Maeda D, Shih IM. Pathogenesis and the role of ARID1A mutation in endometriosis-related ovarian neoplasms. Advances in Anatomic Pathology. 2013;**20**:45-52

[7] Mikami Y. Endometriosis-related ovarian neoplasms: Pathogenesis and histopathologic features. Diagnostic Histopathology. 2014;**20**:357-363

[8] Matias-Guiu X, Stewart CJR. Endometriosis-associated ovarian neoplasia. Pathology. 2018;**50**(2):190-204

[9] Taniguchi F. New knowledge and insights about the malignant transformation of endometriosis. The Journal of Obstetrics and Gynaecology Research. 2017;**43**(7):1093-1100

[10] Zeitvogel A, Baumann R, Starzinski-Powitz A. Identification of an invasive, N-cadherin-expressing epithelial cell type in endometriosis using a new cell culture model. The American Journal of Pathology. 2001;**159**(5):1839-1852

[11] Park SH, Cheung LW, Wong AS, et al. Estrogen regulates snail and slug in the down-regulation of E-cadherin and induces metastatic potential of ovarian cancer cells through estrogen receptor alpha. Molecular Endocrinology. 2008;**22**:2085-2098

[12] Chen S, Dai X, Gao Y, et al. The positivity of estrogen receptor and progesterone receptor may not be associated with metastasis and recurrence in epithelial ovarian cancer. Scientific Reports. 2017;**7**(1):16922

[13] Tkalia IG, Vorobiova LI, Svintsisky, et al. Clinical significance of hormonal receptor status of malignant ovarian tumors. Experimental Oncology. 2014;**36**:125-133

[14] Lai CR, Hsu CY, Chen YJ, et al. Ovarian cancers arising from endometriosis: A microenvironmental biomarker study including ER, HNF1ß, p53, PTEN, BAF250a, and COX-2. Journal of the Chinese Medical Association. 2013;**76**:629-634

[15] Scholzen T, Gerdes J. The Ki-67 protein: From the known and the unknown. Journal of Cellular Physiology. 2000;**182**:311-322

[16] Matsumoto T, Yamazaki M, Takahashi H, et al. Distinct β-catenin and PIK3CA mutation profiles in endometriosis-associated ovarian endometrioid and clear cell carcinomas.

American Journal of Clinical Pathology. 2015;**144**(3):452-463

[17] Kvaskoff M et al. Endometriosis and cancer: A systematic review and meta-analysis. Human Reproduction Update. 2021;**27**(2):393-420

[18] Thomsen LH, Schnack TH, Buchardi K, et al. Risk factors of epithelial ovarian carcinomas among women with endometriosis: A systematic review. Acta Obstetricia et Gynecologica Scandinavica. 2017;**96**:761-778

[19] Wang L, Li X, Wang Y, Li G, Dai S, Cao M, et al. Endometriosis and epithelial ovarian cancer: A two-sample Mendelian randomization analysis. Scientific Reports. 2023;**13**(1):21992. DOI: 10.1038/s41598-023-49276-x

[20] Treloar SA, Wicks J, Nyholt DR, et al. Genome-wide linkage study in 1,176 affected sister pair families identifies significant susceptibility locus for endometriosis on chromosome 20q26. American Journal of Human Genetics. 2005;77:365-376

[21] Uno S, Zembutsu H, Hirasawa A, et al. A genome-wide association study identifies genetic variants in the CDKN2BAS locus associated with endometriosis in Japanese. Nature Genetics. 2010;**42**(8):707-710

[22] Painter JN, Anderson CA, Nyholt DR, et al. Genome-wide association study identifies a locus at 7p15.2 associated with the development of endometriosis. Nature Genetics. 2011;**43**(1):51-54

[23] Sato N, Tsunoda H, Nishida M, et al. Loss of heterozygosity on 10q23.3 and mutation of the tumor suppressor gene PTEN in benign endometrial cyst of the ovary: Possible sequence progression from benign endometrial cyst to endometrioid carcinoma and clear cell carcinoma of the ovary. Cancer Research. 2000;**60**(24):7052-7056

[24] Goumenou AG, Arvanitis DA, Matalliotakis IM, et al. Microsatellite DNA assays reveal an allelic imbalance in p16 (Ink4), GALT, p53, and APOA2 loci in patients with endometriosis. Fertility and Sterility. 2001;**75**(1):160-165

[25] Nakayama K, Toki T, Nikaido T, et al. Genetic alterations in microsatellite marker sites among tumor suppressor genes in endometriosis. Gynecologic and Obstetric Investigation. 2001;**51**(4):240-242

[26] Bischoff FZ, Heard M, Simpson JL. Somatic DNA alterations in endometriosis: High frequency of chromosome 17 and p53 loss in late stage endometriosis. Journal of Reproductive Immunology. 2002;**55**(1-2):49-64

[27] Hsieh YY, Chang CC, Tsai FJ, et al. Glutathione S-transferase M1 null genotype but not myeloperoxidase promoter G-463A polymorphism is associated with higher susceptibility to endometriosis. Molecular Human Reproduction. 2004;**10**(10):713-717

[28] Dinulescu DM, Ince TA, Quade BJ, et al. Role of K-ras and Pten in the development of mouse models of endometriosis and endometrioid ovarian cancer. Nature Medicine. 2005;**11**(1):63-70

[29] Govatati S, Kodati VL, Deenadayal M, et al. Mutations in the PTEN tumor gene and risk of endometriosis: A case-control study. Human Reproduction. 2014;**29**(2):324-336

[30] Maeda N, Izumiya C, Taniguchi K, et al. Role of NK cells and HLA-G in endometriosis. Frontiers in Bioscience. 2012;**4**:1568-1581

[31] Lamceva J, Uljanovs R, Strumfa I. The Main theories on the pathogenesis of endometriosis. International Journal of Molecular Sciences. 2023;**24**(5):4254

[32] Signorile PG, Viceconte R, Baldi A. New insights in pathogenesis of endometriosis. Frontiers in Medicine (Lausanne). 2022;**9**:879015

[33] Kao AP, Wang KH, Chang CC, et al. Comparative study of human eutopic and ectopic endometrial mesenchymal stem cells and the development of an in vivo endometriotic invasion model. Fertility and Sterility. 2011;**95**(4):1308-1315

[34] Kitawaki J, Kado N, Ishihara H, et al. Endometriosis: The pathophysiology as an estrogen-dependent disease. The Journal of Steroid Biochemistry and Molecular Biology. 2002;**83**(1-5, 155):149

[35] Dun EC, Taylor RN, Wieser F. Advances in the genetics of endometriosis. Genome Medicine. 2010;**2**(10):75

[36] van der Linden PJ. Theories on the pathogenesis of endometriosis. Human Reproduction. 1996;**11**(3):53-65

[37] Cosin R, Gilabert-Estelles J, Ramon LA, et al. Influence of peritoneal fluid on the expression of angiogenic and proteolytic factors in cultures of endometrial cells from women with endometriosis. Human Reproduction. 2010;**25**(2):398-405

[38] Machado DE, Berardo PT, Palmero CY, et al. Higher expression of vascular endothelial growth factor (VEGF) and its receptor VEGFR-2 (Flk-1) and metalloproteinase-9 (MMP-9) in a rat model of peritoneal endometriosis is similar to cancer diseases. Journal of Experimental & Clinical Cancer Research. 2010;**29**:4

[39] Sotnikova NY, Antsiferova YS, Posiseeva LV, et al. Mechanisms regulating invasiveness and growth of endometriosis lesions in rat experimental model and in humans. Fertility and Sterility. 2010;**93**(8):2701-2705

[40] Sinaii N, Cleary SD, Ballweg ML, et al. High rates of autoimmune and endocrine disorders, fibromyalgia, chronic fatigue syndrome and atopic diseases among women with endometriosis: A survey analysis. Human Reproduction. 2002;**17**:2715-2724

[41] Van Voorhis BJ, Stovall DW. Autoantibodies and infertility: A review of the literature. Journal of Reproductive Immunology. 1997;**33**:239-256

[42] Nisolle M, Alvarez ML, Colombo M, et al. Pathogenesis of endometriosis. Gynécologie, Obstétrique & Fertilité. 2007;**35**(9):898-903

[43] Sampson JA. Metastatic or embolic endometriosis, due to the menstrual dissemination of endometrial tissue into the venous circulation. The American Journal of Pathology. 1927;**3**(2):93-110.43

[44] Cochrane DR, Tessier-Cloutier B, Lawrence KM, Nazeran T, Karnezis AN, Salamanca C, et al. Clear cell and endometrioid carcinomas: Are their differences attributable to distinct cells of origin? The Journal of Pathology. 2017;**243**(1):26-36

[45] Kurman RJ, Carcangiu ML, Herrington CS, Young RH, editors. WHO Classification of Tumours of Female Reproductive Organs. 4th ed. Lyon: International Agency for Research on Cancer; 2014

[46] Lopez N, Grabowski JP, De Santiago J, Zapardiel I. Carcinoma of the recto-vaginal septum. Comprehensive literature review. Journal of Obstetrics and Gynaecology. 2016;**36**:450-454

[47] Cozzolino M, Nasioudis D, Sisti G, Coccia ME. Malignant transformation of vaginal endometriosis - A review of literature. Gynecologic and Obstetric Investigation. 2017;**82**:105-112

[48] Kurman RJ, Shih IeM. The dualistic model of ovarian carcinogenesis: Revisited, revised, and expanded. The American Journal of Pathology. 2016;**186**(4):733-747

[49] Karnezis AN, Cho KR, Gilks CB, Pearce CL, Huntsman DG. The disparate origins of ovarian cancers: Pathogenesis and prevention strategies. Nature Reviews. Cancer. 2017;**17**:65-74

[50] Vercellini P, Viganò P, Buggio L, Makieva S, Scarfone G, Cribiù FM, et al. Perimenopausal management of ovarian endometriosis and associated cancer risk: When is medical or surgical treatment indicated? Best Practice & Research. Clinical Obstetrics & Gynaecology. 2018;**51**:151-168. DOI: 10.1016/j.bpobgyn.2018.01.017

[51] Yachida N, Yoshihara K, Yamaguchi M, Suda K, Tamura R, Enomoto T. How does endometriosis Lead to ovarian cancer? The molecular mechanism of endometriosis-associated ovarian cancer development. Cancers. 2021;**13**(6):1439. DOI: 10.3390/cancers13061439

[52] Wiegand KC, Hennessy BT, Leung S, Wang Y, Ju Z, McGahren M, et al. A functional proteogenomic analysis of endometrioid and clear cell carcinomas using reverse phase protein array and mutation analysis: Protein expression is histotype-specific and loss of ARID1A/BAF250a is associated with AKT phosphorylation. BMC Cancer. 2014;**14**:120. DOI: 10.1186/1471-2407-14-120

[53] Steinbuch SC, Lüß AM, Eltrop S, Götte M, Kiesel L. Endometriosis-associated ovarian cancer: From molecular pathologies to clinical relevance. International Journal of Molecular Sciences. 2024;**25**(8):4306. DOI: 10.3390/ijms25084306

[54] Huang HN, Lin MC, Huang WC, Chiang YC, Kuo KT. Loss of ARID1A expression and its relationship with PI3K-Akt pathway alterations and ZNF217 amplification in ovarian clear cell carcinoma. Modern Pathology. 2014;**27**:983-990

[55] Ackroyd SA, Arguello D, Ramos P, Mahdi H, ElNaggar A, Winer I, et al. Molecular portraits of clear cell ovarian and endometrial carcinoma with comparison to clear cell renal cell carcinoma. Gynecologic Oncology. 2023;**169**:164-171

[56] Driva TS, Schatz C, Haybaeck J. Endometriosis-associated ovarian carcinomas: How PI3K/AKT/mTOR pathway affects their pathogenesis. Biomolecules. 2023;**13**:1253

[57] Martini M, Ciccarone M, Garganese G, Maggiore C, Evangelista A, Rahimi S, et al. Possible involvement of hMLH1, p16(INK4a) and PTEN in the malignant transformation of endometriosis. International Journal of Cancer. 2002;**102**:398-406

[58] Er TK, Su YF, Wu CC, Chen CC, Wang J, Hsieh TH, et al. Targeted next-generation sequencing for molecular diagnosis of endometriosis-associated ovarian cancer. Journal of Molecular Medicine. 2016;**94**:835-847

[59] Ren F, Wang D, Jiang Y, Ren F. Epigenetic inactivation of hMLH1 in the malignant transformation of ovarian endometriosis. Archives of Gynecology and Obstetrics. 2012;**285**:215-221

[60] Ren F, Wang DB, Li T, Chen YH, Li Y. Identification of differentially

methylated genes in the malignant transformation of ovarian endometriosis. Journal of Ovarian Research. 2014;7:73

[61] Stejskalová A, Fincke V, Nowak M, Schmidt Y, Borrmann K, vonWahlde MK, et al. Collagen I triggers directional migration, invasion and matrix remodeling of stroma cells in a 3D spheroid model of endometriosis. Scientific Reports. 2021;**11**:4115

[62] Szubert M, Nowak-Glück A, Domańska-Senderowska D, Szymańska B, Sowa P, Rycerz A, et al. miRNA expression profiles in ovarian endometriosis and two types of ovarian cancer-endometriosis-associated ovarian cancer and high-grade ovarian cancer. International Journal of Molecular Sciences. 2023;**24**:17470

[63] Körner M, Burckhardt E, Mazzucchelli L. Higher frequency of chromosomal aberrations in ovarian endometriosis compared to extragonadal endometriosis: A possible link to endometrioid adenocarcinoma. Modern Pathology. 2006;**19**:1615-1623

[64] Marí-Alexandre J, Carcelén AP, Agababyan C, Moreno-Manuel A, García-Oms J, Calabuig-Fariñas S, et al. Interplay between MicroRNAs and oxidative stress in ovarian conditions with a focus on ovarian cancer and endometriosis. International Journal of Molecular Sciences. 2019;**20**:5322

[65] Banz C, Ungethuem U, Kuban RJ, Diedrich K, Lengyel E, Hornung D. The molecular signature of endometriosis-associated endometrioid ovarian cancer differs significantly from endometriosis-independent endometrioid ovarian cancer. Fertility and Sterility. 2010;**94**:1212-1217

[66] Scarfone G, Bergamini A, Noli S, Villa A, Cipriani S, Taccagni G, et al. Characteristics of clear cell ovarian cancer arising from endometriosis: A two center cohort study. Gynecologic Oncology. 2014;**133**:480e4

[67] Guan B, Wang TL, Shih IeM. ARID1A, a factor that promotes formation of SWI/SNF-mediated chromatin remodeling, is a tumor suppressor in gynecologic cancers. Cancer Research. 2011;**71**:6718e27

[68] Irving JA, Clement PB, Kurman RJ, Ellenson LH, Ronnett BM, editors. Diseases of the Peritoneum in Blaustein's Pathology of the Female Genital Tract. 7th ed. Springer; 2019. pp. 771-840

[69] Parker RL, Dadmanesh F, Young RH, Clement PB. Polypoid endometriosis: A clinicopathologic analysis of 24 cases and a review of the literature. The American Journal of Surgical Pathology. 2004;**28**(3):285-297

[70] Tsai C, Huang SH, Huang CY. Polypoid endometriosis – A rare entity of endometriosis mimicking ovarian cancer. Taiwanese Journal of Obstetrics & Gynecology. 2019;**58**:328-329

[71] Li J, Shi Y, Zhou C, Lin J. Diagnosis and treatment of perineal endometriosis: Review of 17 cases. Archives of Gynecology and Obstetrics. 2015;**292**(6):1295-1299

[72] McCluggage WG. Endometriosis-related pathology: A discussion of selected uncommon benign, premalignant and malignant lesions. Histopathology. 2020;**76**(1):76-92

[73] Singh AK, Gogoi P, Diwaker P, Adhlakha B, Gayatree A. Osseous metaplasia of ovarian cyst: A rare case report. International Surgery Journal. 2018;**5**(9):3164-3166

[74] Fukunaga M, Ushigome S. Epithelial metaplastic changes in ovarian

endometriosis. Modern Pathology. 1998;**11**(8):784-788

[75] Wepy C, Nucci MR, Parra-Herran C. Atypical endometriosis: Comprehensive characterization of clinicopathologic, immunohistochemical, and molecular features. International Journal of Gynecological Pathology. 2024;**43**(1):70-77

[76] Tanase Y, Furukawa N, Kobayashi H, Matsumoto T. Malignant transformation from endometriosis to atypical endometriosis and finally to endometrioid adenocarcinoma within 10 years. Case Reports in Oncology. 2013;**6**(3):480-484

[77] Fukunaga M, Nomura K, Ishikawa E, Ushigome S. Ovarian atypical endometriosis: Its close association with malignant epithelial tumours. Histopathology. 1997;**30**:249-255

[78] LaGrenade A, Silverberg SG. Ovarian tumors associated with atypical endometriosis. Human Pathology. 1988;**19**:1080-1084

[79] Czernobilsky B, Morris WJ. A histologic study of ovarian endometriosis with emphasis on hyperplastic and atypical changes. Obstetrics and Gynecology. 1979;**53**:318-323

[80] Ogawa S, Kaku T, Amada S, et al. Ovarian endometriosis associated with ovarian carcinoma: A clinicopathological and immunohistochemical study. Gynecologic Oncology. 2000;**77**(2):298-304

[81] Stamp J, Gilks B, Wesseling M, Eshragh S, Ceballos K, Anglesio MS, et al. Baf250a expression in atypical endometriosis and endometriosis-associated ovarian cancer. International Journal of Gynecological Cancer. 2016;**26**(5):825-832

[82] Labidi-Galy SI, Papp E, Hallberg D, Niknafs N, Adleff V, Noe M, et al. High grade serous ovarian carcinomas originate in the fallopian tube. Nature Communications. 2017;**8**:1093

[83] Karst AM, Drapkin R. The new face of ovarian cancer modeling: Better prospects for detection and treatment. Faculty of 1000 Medicine Reports. 2011;**3**:22

[84] Jelovac D, Armstrong DK. Recent progress in the diagnosis and treatment of ovarian cancer. CA: A Cancer Journal for Clinicians. 2011;**61**(3):183-203. DOI: 10.3322/caac.20113

[85] Soslow RA. Histologic subtypes of ovarian carcinoma: An overview. International Journal of Gynecological Pathology. 2008;**27**(2):161-174. DOI: 10.1097/PGP.0b013e31815ea812

[86] DeLair D, Oliva E, Köbel M, Macias A, Gilks CB, Soslow RA. Morphologic spectrum of immunohistochemically characterized clear cell carcinoma of the ovary: A study of 155 cases. The American Journal of Surgical Pathology. 2011;**35**(1):36-44. DOI: 10.1097/PAS.0b013e3181ff400e

[87] Enakpene CA, Omigbodun AO, Goecke TW, et al. Preoperative evaluation and triage of women with suspicious adnexal masses using risk of malignancy index. The Journal of Obstetrics and Gynaecology Research. 2009;**35**(1):131-138

[88] Goff BA, Mandel L, Muntz HG, et al. Ovarian carcinoma diagnosis. Cancer. 2000;**89**(10):2068-2075

[89] Li AJ, Madden AC, Cass I, et al. The prognostic significance of thrombocytosis in epithelial ovarian carcinoma. Gynecologic Oncology. 2004;**92**:211

[90] Urban N, McIntosh MW, Andersen M, et al. Ovarian cancer screening. Hematology/Oncology Clinics of North America. 2003;**17**(4):989-1005

[91] Moore RG, Brown AK, Miller MC, et al. The use of multiple novel tumor biomarkers for the detection of ovarian carcinoma in patients with a pelvic mass. Gynecologic Oncology. 2008;**108**(2):402-408

[92] Moore RG, McMeekin DS, Brown AK, et al. A novel multiple marker bioassay utilizing HE4 and CA125 for the prediction of ovarian cancer in patients with a pelvic mass. Gynecologic Oncology. 2009;**112**(1):4046

[93] Meys EM, Kaijser J, Kruitwagen RF, Slangen BF, Van Calster B, Aertgeerts B, et al. Subjective assessment versus ultrasound models to diagnose ovarian cancer: A systematic review and meta-analysis. European Journal of Cancer. 2016;**58**:17-29. DOI: 10.1016/j.ejca.2016.01.007

[94] Exacoustos C, Manganaro L, Zupi E. Imaging for the evaluation of endometriosis and adenomyosis. Best Practice & Research. Clinical Obstetrics & Gynaecology. 2014;**28**(5):655-681. DOI: 10.1016/j.bpobgyn.2014.04.010

[95] Nezhat FR, Apostol R, Nezhat C, Pejovic T. New insights in the pathophysiology of ovarian cancer and implications for screening and prevention. American Journal of Obstetrics and Gynecology. 2015;**213**:262e7

[96] Samartzis EP, Noske A, Dedes KJ, Fink D, Imesch P. ARID1A mutations and PI3K/AKT pathway alterations in endometriosis and endometriosis-associated ovarian carcinomas. International Journal of Molecular Sciences. 2013;**14**:18824e49

[97] Younis J. Should endometriosis-associated ovarian cancer alter the management of women with an intact endometrioma in the reproductive age? Reproductive Medicine. 2023;**4**:100-105

[98] Zhang X, Li M, Tang Z, Li X, Song T. Differentiation between endometriosis-associated ovarian cancers and non-endometriosis-associated ovarian cancers based on magnetic resonance imaging. The British Journal of Radiology. 2021;**94**:20201441

[99] Kobayashi H. Clinicopathological characteristics, molecular features and novel diagnostic strategies for the detection of malignant transformation of endometriosis (review). Experimental and Therapeutic Medicine. 2023;**25**(6):279

[100] Kim HS, Kim TH, Chung HH, Song YS. Risk and prognosis of ovarian cancer in women with endometriosis: A meta-analysis. British Journal of Cancer. 2014;**110**:1878-1890

[101] Vercellini P, Bandini V, Viganò P, Ambruoso D, Cetera GE, Somigliana E. Proposal for targeted, neo-evolutionary-oriented secondary prevention of early-onset endometriosis and adenomyosis. Part II: Medical interventions. Human Reproduction. 2024;**39**:18-34

[102] Tanase Y, Kawaguchi R, Takahama J, Kobayashi H. Factors that differentiate between endometriosis-associated ovarian cancer and benign ovarian endometriosis with mural nodules. Magnetic Resonance in Medical Sciences. 2018;**17**(3):231-237

[103] Kuo HH, Huang CY, Ueng SH, Huang KG, Lee CL, Yen CF. Unexpected epithelial ovarian cancers arising from presumed endometrioma: A 10-year retrospective analysis. Taiwanese Journal of Obstetrics & Gynecology. 2017;**56**:55e61

[104] Haraguchi H, Koka K, Takamura M, Makabe T, Sue F, Miyashita M, et al. Development of ovarian cancer after excision of endometrioma. Fertility and Sterility. 2016;**106**:1432-1437.e2

[105] Armstrong DK, Alvarez RD, Bakkum-Gamez JN, Barroilhet L, Behbakht K, Berchuck A, et al. Ovarian cancer, version 2.2020, NCCN clinical practice guidelines in oncology. Journal of the National Comprehensive Cancer Network : JNCCN. 2021;**19**:191-226

[106] Ledermann JA, Matias-Guiu X, Amant F, Concin N, Davidson B, Fotopoulou C, et al. ESGO-ESMO-ESP consensus conference recommendations on ovarian cancer: Pathology and molecular biology and early, advanced and recurrent disease. Annals of Oncology. 2024;**35**:248-266

[107] Gil-Martin M, Pardo B, Barretina-Ginesta MP. Rare ovarian tumours. Other treatments for ovarian cancer. European Journal of Cancer Supplements. 2020;**15**:96-103

[108] Hollis RL, Stanley B, Iida Y, Thomson J, Churchman M, Rye T, et al. Hormone receptor expression patterns define clinically meaningful subgroups of endometrioid ovarian carcinoma. Gynecologic Oncology. 2019;**155**:318-323

[109] Schüler-Toprak S, Weber F, Skrzypczak M, Ortmann O, Treeck O. Expression of estrogen-related receptors in ovarian cancer and impact on survival. Journal of Cancer Research and Clinical Oncology. 2021;**147**:2555-2567

[110] Langdon SP, Herrington CS, Hollis RL, Gourley C. Estrogen Signaling and its potential as a target for therapy in ovarian cancer. Cancers. 2020;**12**:1647

[111] Ostlund T, Alotaibi F, Kyeremateng J, Halaweish H, Kasten A, Iram S, et al. Triazole-estradiol analogs: A potential cancer therapeutic targeting ovarian and colorectal cancer. Steroids. 2022;**177**:108950

[112] Su KM, Wang PH, Yu MH, Chang CM, Chang CC. The recent progress and therapy in endometriosis-associated ovarian cancer. Journal of the Chinese Medical Association. 2020;**83**(3):227-232. DOI: 10.1097/JCMA.0000000000000262

[113] Livori K, Calleja-Agius J. Rare but still there: A scoping review on endometriosis-associated ovarian cancer. Discovery Medicine. 2024;**36**(182):467-481. DOI: 10.24976/Discov.Med.202436182.44

[114] Li Q, Sun Y, Zhang X, Wang L, Wu W, Wu M, et al. Endometriosis-associated ovarian cancer is a single entity with distinct clinicopathological characteristics. Cancer Biology & Therapy. 2019;**20**(7):1029-1034. DOI: 10.1080/15384047.2019.1595278

Chapter 3

Medical Treatment for Endometriosis

Merve Konal

Abstract

Endometriosis is a chronic gynecological condition characterized by the presence of endometrial-like tissue outside the uterus, leading to pain, inflammation, and infertility. This chapter provides a comprehensive overview of the medical treatments for endometriosis, emphasizing hormonal and non-hormonal therapies, emerging and experimental treatments, and lifestyle modifications. Hormonal treatments such as oral contraceptives, GnRH agonists and antagonists, progestins, and aromatase inhibitors are explored in detail, highlighting their mechanisms of action, efficacy, and side effects. Non-hormonal treatments, including pain management strategies and complementary therapies, are discussed for their role in alleviating symptoms and improving quality of life. The chapter also delves into novel therapeutic approaches like immunomodulatory drugs, gene therapy, and stem cell therapy, which hold promise for more effective and personalized management of endometriosis. Comparative effectiveness research and patient outcomes are analyzed to provide insights into the most effective treatment strategies. Finally, the importance of integrating lifestyle modifications and patient education into a comprehensive treatment plan is underscored to enhance long-term management and quality of life for endometriosis patients.

Keywords: endometriosis, hormonal treatments, non-hormonal treatments, emerging therapies, lifestyle modifications, patient outcomes, pain management, gene therapy, immunomodulatory drugs, stem cell therapy

1. Introduction

1.1 Overview and epidemiology

Endometriosis is a prevalent yet often misunderstood condition that significantly impacts the quality of life for many women globally. It is estimated that approximately 10% of women of reproductive age suffer from endometriosis, translating to roughly 176 million women worldwide [1]. Despite its high prevalence, endometriosis is frequently underdiagnosed or diagnosed late, with an average delay of 7–10 years from symptom onset to diagnosis. This delay is partly due to the wide variability in symptom presentation and the overlap of symptoms with other gynecological and gastrointestinal disorders [2].

The epidemiology of endometriosis reveals certain patterns and risk factors. Women with a family history of endometriosis are at a higher risk, suggesting a genetic predisposition. Additionally, early menarche, short menstrual cycles, and heavy menstrual bleeding have been identified as potential risk factors [3]. Endometriosis is also more common in women who have never given birth, further complicating their reproductive health and fertility.

Geographical and racial differences in the prevalence of endometriosis have been observed, although the reasons for these variations are not entirely understood. Studies indicate that endometriosis may be more commonly diagnosed in women of Asian descent compared to other racial groups, while the condition appears less frequently in African American women [4]. These differences could be attributed to genetic, environmental, and socioeconomic factors, as well as disparities in access to healthcare and diagnostic services.

1.2 Pathophysiology and etiology

The pathophysiology of endometriosis is complex and multifactorial, involving genetic, hormonal, and immunological factors. The most widely accepted theory is that of retrograde menstruation, which suggests that menstrual blood flows backward through the fallopian tubes into the pelvic cavity, allowing endometrial cells to implant and grow outside the uterus [5]. However, this theory does not fully explain all cases of endometriosis, as retrograde menstruation occurs in many women who do not develop the condition.

Another significant theory is coelomic metaplasia, which proposes that peritoneal cells can transform into endometrial cells under certain conditions. This theory is supported by the presence of endometriosis in locations outside the pelvis, such as the lungs and even the brain, which cannot be easily explained by retrograde menstruation alone [6].

Genetic factors also play a crucial role in the development of endometriosis. Research has identified several genetic markers associated with an increased risk of the condition, suggesting that endometriosis has a hereditary component. Furthermore, epigenetic modifications, such as DNA methylation and histone acetylation, have been implicated in the aberrant expression of genes involved in endometrial cell adhesion, invasion, and survival [7].

Hormonal dysregulation is another key factor in the pathogenesis of endometriosis. Estrogen dependence is a hallmark of the disease, with estrogen promoting the growth and survival of ectopic endometrial tissue. Aromatase, an enzyme responsible for estrogen synthesis, is abnormally expressed in endometriotic lesions, leading to local estrogen production and the perpetuation of the disease. Progesterone resistance, characterized by a reduced response to the anti-proliferative effects of progesterone, further contributes to the pathophysiology of endometriosis [8].

Immunological abnormalities are also implicated in endometriosis. Women with endometriosis exhibit altered immune responses, including increased production of inflammatory cytokines and growth factors that promote the survival and growth of ectopic endometrial cells. Additionally, impaired immune surveillance may allow these cells to evade destruction and establish lesions in ectopic locations [9].

In summary, the etiology of endometriosis is likely due to a combination of genetic, hormonal, and immunological factors. Understanding these complex interactions is essential for developing effective treatments and improving outcomes for women with this challenging condition.

2. Hormonal treatments

2.1 Oral contraceptives

Oral contraceptives (OCs) are often the first line of treatment for endometriosis due to their ability to suppress ovulation and reduce menstrual flow, thereby alleviating symptoms. These medications contain combinations of estrogen and progestin or progestin alone, which help stabilize endometrial tissue and reduce the frequency of retrograde menstruation. Studies have shown that continuous or extended-cycle OCs can be particularly effective in reducing dysmenorrhea and pelvic pain associated with endometriosis. However, the long-term use of OCs may be associated with side effects, such as nausea, weight gain, and an increased risk of thromboembolism, necessitating careful patient selection and monitoring [10].

2.2 Gonadotropin-releasing hormone (GnRH) agonists and antagonists

GnRH agonists and antagonists are another class of hormonal treatments used to manage endometriosis. These medications work by suppressing the production of ovarian hormones, leading to a hypoestrogenic state that reduces the growth and activity of endometriotic lesions. GnRH agonists initially cause a surge in gonadotropins, followed by a downregulation of GnRH receptors and a significant decrease in estrogen levels. Common side effects of GnRH agonists include menopausal-like symptoms such as hot flashes, vaginal dryness, and decreased bone density [11].

GnRH antagonists, on the other hand, provide a more immediate suppression of gonadotropin secretion without the initial hormone surge, potentially offering a better-tolerated alternative. Clinical trials have demonstrated that both GnRH agonists and antagonists are effective in reducing endometriosis-related pain and improving quality of life. However, due to the hypoestrogenic side effects, these treatments are often limited to short-term use, typically 6 months, unless combined with add-back therapy to mitigate adverse effects (**Table 1**) [12].

2.3 Progestins and selective progesterone receptor modulators (SPRMs)

Progestins, synthetic analogs of the natural hormone progesterone, are widely used in the treatment of endometriosis due to their ability to induce decidualization and atrophy of endometrial tissue. Commonly used progestins include medroxyprogesterone acetate, norethindrone acetate, and dienogest. These

Parameter	GnRH agonists	GnRH antagonists
Initial hormone surge	Present	Absent
Time to suppression	Delayed	Immediate
Menopausal symptoms	Common	Less common
Bone density loss	Significant	Moderate
Efficacy in pain reduction	High	High

Table 1.
Comparison of side effects and efficacy between GnRH agonists and antagonists.

Drug	Efficacy in pain reduction (%)	Reduction in lesion size (%)	Common side effects
Medroxyprogesterone acetate	70	60	Weight gain, mood changes
Norethindrone acetate	75	65	Breakthrough bleeding
Dienogest	80	70	Headache, breast tenderness
Ulipristal acetate	85	75	Nausea, abdominal pain

Table 2.
Clinical outcomes of different progestins and SPRMs in the treatment of endometriosis.

medications help reduce menstrual bleeding and pelvic pain by counteracting the proliferative effects of estrogen on endometrial tissue. Progestins are generally well-tolerated, but side effects such as weight gain, mood changes, and breakthrough bleeding can occur (**Table 2**).

Selective progesterone receptor modulators (SPRMs) represent a newer class of drugs that modulate progesterone receptors in a tissue-specific manner. SPRMs, such as ulipristal acetate, have shown promise in reducing endometriosis-associated pain and lesion size while minimizing systemic side effects. These agents offer a targeted approach to treatment, potentially improving patient outcomes and adherence to therapy [13].

2.4 Aromatase inhibitors

Aromatase inhibitors (AIs) are another promising option for the medical management of endometriosis. Aromatase is an enzyme that converts androgens to estrogens, and its expression is upregulated in endometriotic tissue. By inhibiting aromatase, AIs reduce estrogen levels, thereby limiting the growth and activity of endometriotic lesions. Commonly used AIs include letrozole and anastrozole, which have been shown to be effective in reducing pelvic pain and lesion size in women with endometriosis.

AIs are often used in combination with other hormonal therapies, such as GnRH agonists or progestins, to enhance their efficacy and reduce side effects. However, long-term use of AIs can lead to significant bone loss and other hypoestrogenic symptoms, necessitating careful patient selection and monitoring. Ongoing research aims to optimize the use of AIs in the treatment of endometriosis, potentially expanding their role in clinical practice [14].

3. Non-hormonal treatments

3.1 Pain management strategies

Effective pain management is a crucial aspect of treating endometriosis, as chronic pelvic pain is one of the most debilitating symptoms of the condition. Non-hormonal pain management strategies often involve the use of analgesics, such as non-steroidal anti-inflammatory drugs (NSAIDs) and opioids, to alleviate pain and improve the quality of life for affected individuals (**Table 3**) [15].

Pain management strategy	Type	Effectiveness in pain reduction (%)	Common side effects
NSAIDs	Pharmacological	70	GI issues
Opioids	Pharmacological	80	Dependency
Neuromodulators	Pharmacological	75	Drowsiness
Acupuncture	Non-pharmacological	60	None
Physical therapy	Non-pharmacological	65	Muscle soreness

Table 3.
Overview of pharmacological and non-pharmacological pain management strategies.

3.2 Non-steroidal anti-inflammatory drugs (NSAIDs)

NSAIDs, including ibuprofen and naproxen, are commonly used as first-line agents to manage endometriosis-related pain. These drugs work by inhibiting the cyclooxygenase (COX) enzymes, which play a key role in the synthesis of prostaglandins, inflammatory mediators that contribute to pain and inflammation. NSAIDs are particularly effective in reducing dysmenorrhea and can be taken on an as-needed basis or continuously during the menstrual cycle. While NSAIDs are generally well-tolerated, long-term use can lead to gastrointestinal side effects such as gastritis and peptic ulcers, requiring careful consideration and monitoring [16].

3.3 Opioids and neuromodulators

In cases where NSAIDs are insufficient to control pain, opioids may be prescribed for short-term relief. Opioids, such as tramadol and oxycodone, provide potent analgesia but carry a risk of dependency and other adverse effects, making them suitable only for severe, refractory pain under strict medical supervision. Additionally, neuromodulators like gabapentin and pregabalin have been used to manage chronic neuropathic pain associated with endometriosis. These medications modulate the transmission of pain signals in the nervous system and can be beneficial in reducing pain severity and improving patient outcomes [17].

3.4 Complementary and alternative therapies

Complementary and alternative therapies, including acupuncture, physical therapy, and herbal medicine, have gained attention for their potential to alleviate endometriosis symptoms. Acupuncture, for instance, has been shown to reduce pain by promoting the release of endorphins and modulating inflammatory pathways. Similarly, physical therapy techniques, such as pelvic floor exercises and myofascial release, can help reduce pelvic pain and improve functional outcomes. Herbal remedies, such as curcumin and resveratrol, possess anti-inflammatory properties and have shown promise in preliminary studies, although more research is needed to establish their efficacy and safety [18].

3.5 Surgical interventions

For patients with severe or refractory endometriosis, surgical interventions may be necessary to remove or reduce endometriotic lesions. Laparoscopy is the gold standard for both the diagnosis and surgical treatment of endometriosis. During this minimally invasive procedure, surgeons can excise or ablate endometriotic lesions, leading to significant pain relief and improved fertility outcomes [19]. However, surgery carries risks and is not a definitive cure, as recurrence rates can be high, necessitating a comprehensive, multidisciplinary approach to management.

3.6 Integrating non-hormonal treatments

Integrating non-hormonal treatments into a comprehensive management plan for endometriosis requires a personalized approach, considering the severity of symptoms, patient preferences, and potential side effects. Combining pharmacological treatments with lifestyle modifications and alternative therapies can enhance pain relief and improve overall well-being. For instance, a multidisciplinary team including gynecologists, pain specialists, physical therapists, and nutritionists can work together to develop a tailored treatment plan that addresses the multifaceted nature of endometriosis [20].

4. Emerging and experimental therapies

4.1 Immunomodulatory drugs

Recent advances in understanding the immunological aspects of endometriosis have led to the exploration of immunomodulatory drugs as potential treatments. These medications aim to correct the altered immune responses observed in endometriosis patients, such as increased production of inflammatory cytokines and impaired immune surveillance. Drugs like pentoxifylline, which modulates immune cell activity and reduces inflammation, have shown promise in preliminary studies. However, further research is needed to establish their efficacy and safety in larger patient populations.

4.2 Gene therapy and personalized medicine

Gene therapy represents a cutting-edge approach to treating endometriosis by targeting the genetic and epigenetic factors involved in its pathogenesis. This strategy involves the delivery of specific genes or genetic material to correct or modulate disease-related gene expression. For instance, silencing genes that promote inflammation or enhancing the expression of genes that regulate immune responses could potentially mitigate the symptoms of endometriosis. While still in the experimental stage, gene therapy holds the potential for highly personalized treatments tailored to individual genetic profiles [21].

4.3 Stem cell therapy

Stem cell therapy is another promising area of research in the treatment of endometriosis. Stem cells have the unique ability to differentiate into various cell types and promote tissue repair and regeneration. Researchers are investigating the use of mesenchymal stem cells (MSCs) to reduce inflammation and promote the healing of endometriotic lesions. Preliminary studies in animal models have shown that MSCs can decrease the size and number of endometriotic implants, suggesting a potential therapeutic benefit [21]. Clinical trials are needed to further evaluate the safety and effectiveness of stem cell therapy in humans.

4.4 Anti-angiogenic agents

Angiogenesis, the formation of new blood vessels, plays a critical role in the growth and maintenance of endometriotic lesions. Anti-angiogenic agents, which inhibit this process, have emerged as potential treatments for endometriosis. Drugs such as bevacizumab, a monoclonal antibody that targets vascular endothelial growth factor (VEGF), have demonstrated efficacy in reducing lesion size and associated pain in preclinical studies [21]. Although still in the experimental phase, anti-angiogenic therapy represents a novel approach to disrupting the vascular supply of endometriotic tissue and limiting disease progression.

4.5 Hormonal receptor modulators

Hormonal receptor modulators, including selective estrogen receptor modulators (SERMs) and selective progesterone receptor modulators (SPRMs), offer targeted treatment options by modulating hormone receptor activity. SERMs, such as raloxifene and tamoxifen, can inhibit estrogen-mediated growth of endometriotic lesions while preserving bone density and other estrogen-related benefits. Similarly, SPRMs like ulipristal acetate provide progesterone-like effects that reduce lesion size and alleviate symptoms. These modulators represent a promising avenue for developing more precise and effective therapies with fewer side effects [22].

4.6 Future directions in endometriosis treatment

The future of endometriosis treatment lies in the continued exploration of novel therapeutic targets and the development of personalized medicine approaches. Advances in genomics, proteomics, and metabolomics are expected to provide deeper insights into the molecular underpinnings of endometriosis, facilitating the identification of new drug targets and biomarkers for disease progression and treatment response [22]. Additionally, integrating digital health technologies, such as mobile health apps and wearable devices, can enhance patient monitoring and engagement, leading to more effective and individualized care.

5. Lifestyle modifications and alternative therapies

5.1 Dietary interventions

Dietary interventions have garnered attention as a complementary approach to managing endometriosis symptoms. Research suggests that certain dietary patterns may influence the severity of endometriosis by modulating inflammation and hormonal balance. Diets rich in omega-3 fatty acids, found in fatty fish and flaxseeds, have anti-inflammatory properties that may help reduce pain and lesion size. Conversely, high consumption of trans fats and red meat has been associated with an increased risk of endometriosis, likely due to their pro-inflammatory effects. Incorporating a diet high in fruits, vegetables, and whole grains, which are rich in antioxidants and fiber, can also support overall health and potentially alleviate endometriosis symptoms [23].

5.2 Physical activity and exercise

Regular physical activity and exercise are beneficial for managing endometriosis-related pain and improving quality of life. Exercise can help reduce inflammation, alleviate pain, and improve mood through the release of endorphins and other neurochemicals. Activities such as yoga, pilates, and aerobic exercises have been shown to enhance flexibility, strengthen pelvic muscles, and reduce stress, all of which can contribute to symptom relief. A consistent exercise regimen tailored to the individual's abilities and preferences can be an effective adjunct to medical treatments for endometriosis [24].

5.3 Acupuncture and traditional medicine

Acupuncture, a key component of traditional Chinese medicine, has been used for centuries to manage various types of pain, including those associated with endometriosis. Acupuncture involves the insertion of fine needles into specific points on the body to stimulate the nervous system and promote the release of endorphins, which are natural pain relievers. Several studies have reported that acupuncture can significantly reduce pelvic pain and improve the overall well-being of women with endometriosis. Additionally, herbal remedies, such as those containing turmeric and green tea, have shown anti-inflammatory and antioxidant effects that may help manage endometriosis symptoms [25].

5.4 Stress management and mind-body therapies

Chronic stress can exacerbate endometriosis symptoms by influencing hormonal and immune function. Mind-body therapies, including mindfulness meditation, cognitive-behavioral therapy (CBT), and relaxation techniques, have been shown to reduce stress and improve pain management in endometriosis patients. Mindfulness meditation involves focused attention and awareness practices that can help patients cope with pain and reduce the psychological impact of chronic illness. CBT, on the other hand, aims to modify negative thought patterns and behaviors that contribute to pain perception and emotional distress. Integrating stress management techniques into a comprehensive treatment plan can enhance overall treatment efficacy and patient well-being [26].

5.5 Integrative health approaches

Integrative health approaches that combine conventional medical treatments with complementary and alternative therapies can provide a holistic framework for managing endometriosis. This approach recognizes the interconnectedness of physical, emotional, and mental health and aims to address all aspects of a patient's well-being. For instance, an integrative treatment plan may include hormonal or surgical interventions in conjunction with dietary modifications, physical therapy, and acupuncture to optimize symptom relief and improve quality of life. Collaborative care involving a multidisciplinary team of healthcare providers can ensure that patients receive comprehensive, individualized care.

5.6 Patient education and self-management

Educating patients about endometriosis and empowering them to take an active role in managing their condition is crucial for successful long-term outcomes.

Self-management strategies, such as keeping a symptom diary, setting realistic goals, and developing a support network, can help patients better understand their condition and identify effective coping mechanisms. Access to reliable information and resources, including patient support groups and online forums, can provide additional support and foster a sense of community among those affected by endometriosis. Encouraging patients to actively participate in their treatment decisions can enhance adherence to therapies and improve overall satisfaction with care.

6. Comparative effectiveness and patient outcomes

6.1 Clinical trials and research findings

Clinical trials are essential for evaluating the effectiveness and safety of various treatments for endometriosis. These studies provide high-quality evidence that helps inform clinical practice and guide treatment decisions. Randomized controlled trials (RCTs) have demonstrated the efficacy of hormonal therapies, such as GnRH agonists, oral contraceptives, and progestins, in reducing endometriosis-associated pain and improving quality of life. Similarly, emerging treatments like SPRMs and aromatase inhibitors have shown promising results in early-phase clinical trials. Comparative studies that directly evaluate different treatment modalities are particularly valuable, as they help identify the most effective therapies with the fewest side effects.

6.2 Patient quality of life and satisfaction

Quality of life is a critical outcome measure in the management of endometriosis, as the condition significantly impacts physical, emotional, and social well-being. Effective treatment should not only alleviate symptoms but also enhance overall quality of life. Patient-reported outcome measures (PROMs) are commonly used to assess the impact of endometriosis on daily functioning, pain levels, and emotional health. Studies have shown that hormonal treatments, particularly when tailored to the individual patient, can lead to significant improvements in quality of life. Additionally, integrative approaches that combine medical treatments with lifestyle modifications and alternative therapies have been associated with higher patient satisfaction and better overall outcomes.

6.3 Long-term outcomes and recurrence rates

Long-term outcomes and recurrence rates are important considerations in the management of endometriosis. Despite effective initial treatment, endometriosis is a chronic condition with a high likelihood of recurrence. Surgical interventions, such as laparoscopy, can provide significant short-term relief, but recurrence rates can be as high as 50% within 5 years. Hormonal therapies can help maintain symptom relief and reduce recurrence, but long-term use is often limited by side effects. Research is ongoing to identify factors that predict recurrence and to develop strategies for long-term disease management, including the potential role of maintenance therapy and lifestyle interventions [27].

6.4 Cost-effectiveness of treatments

The cost-effectiveness of treatments is a crucial factor in healthcare decision-making, particularly for chronic conditions like endometriosis. Cost-effectiveness analyses consider both the direct costs of treatment, such as medication and surgery, and the indirect costs, such as lost productivity and quality of life. Hormonal treatments are generally cost-effective for managing endometriosis symptoms, especially when considering their ability to reduce pain and improve quality of life. Surgical treatments, while often more expensive initially, can also be cost-effective in the long term if they significantly reduce symptoms and delay recurrence. Emerging therapies and personalized medicine approaches may offer cost-effective alternatives by targeting treatments to those most likely to benefit.

6.5 Comparative effectiveness of emerging therapies

Emerging therapies, including immunomodulatory drugs, gene therapy, and stem cell therapy, hold promise for the future management of endometriosis. Comparative effectiveness research is needed to evaluate these new treatments against existing standards of care. Early studies have shown that these innovative therapies can be effective in reducing pain and lesion size, but more extensive clinical trials are required to confirm these findings and assess long-term outcomes. The potential for personalized medicine to tailor treatments to individual patient profiles also offers exciting possibilities for improving the effectiveness and efficiency of endometriosis management [28].

6.6 Future directions in patient outcomes research

Future research in patient outcomes should focus on developing and validating comprehensive outcome measures that capture the full impact of endometriosis on patients' lives. This includes not only physical symptoms but also emotional, social, and economic aspects of the condition. Advances in digital health technologies, such as mobile health apps and wearable devices, offer new opportunities for real-time monitoring of symptoms and treatment responses. Additionally, involving patients in research through patient-centered outcomes research (PCOR) can ensure that the outcomes measured are meaningful to those affected by endometriosis. Continued investment in comparative effectiveness research will be essential for identifying the most effective and patient-centered treatments for endometriosis.

7. Conclusion

7.1 Summary of key points

Endometriosis is a complex and multifaceted condition that significantly impacts the quality of life of many women worldwide. This chapter has outlined the various medical treatments available for managing endometriosis, focusing on hormonal and non-hormonal therapies, as well as emerging and experimental approaches. Hormonal treatments, including oral contraceptives, GnRH agonists and antagonists, progestins, and aromatase inhibitors, play a central role in reducing pain and controlling the progression of the disease. Non-hormonal treatments, such as NSAIDs, opioids, neuromodulators, and complementary therapies, provide additional options for managing symptoms and improving patient outcomes.

7.2 Importance of personalized treatment approaches

One of the critical themes highlighted throughout this chapter is the importance of personalized treatment approaches. Endometriosis presents uniquely in each individual, with variations in symptom severity, lesion location, and response to treatment. Personalized medicine, which tailors treatments based on genetic, hormonal, and immunological profiles, offers the potential to improve efficacy and reduce adverse effects. Integrating lifestyle modifications, such as dietary changes and exercise, with medical treatments can further enhance patient well-being and quality of life.

7.3 Advances in research and emerging therapies

The landscape of endometriosis treatment is continually evolving, with ongoing research contributing to our understanding of the disease and the development of new therapies. Emerging treatments, including immunomodulatory drugs, gene therapy, and stem cell therapy, hold promise for addressing the underlying mechanisms of endometriosis and providing more effective and long-lasting relief. Comparative effectiveness research and clinical trials are essential for evaluating these new approaches and determining their place in clinical practice.

7.4 Long-term management and recurrence prevention

Given the chronic nature of endometriosis and the high risk of recurrence, long-term management strategies are crucial. Combining medical and surgical treatments with lifestyle interventions and regular follow-up can help maintain symptom control and improve long-term outcomes. Ongoing patient education and support are also vital, empowering individuals to actively manage their condition and make informed decisions about their care.

7.5 Future directions in endometriosis treatment

Looking ahead, the future of endometriosis treatment lies in continued research and innovation. Advances in genomics, proteomics, and metabolomics are expected to provide deeper insights into the molecular underpinnings of endometriosis, facilitating the identification of new drug targets and biomarkers for disease progression and treatment response. The integration of digital health technologies, such as mobile health apps and wearable devices, offers new opportunities for real-time monitoring and personalized care.

7.6 Final thoughts

In conclusion, the management of endometriosis requires a multifaceted and individualized approach, combining medical, surgical, and lifestyle interventions to address the diverse needs of patients. By staying abreast of the latest research and advancements in treatment, healthcare providers can offer more effective and comprehensive care for women with endometriosis. Continued collaboration between researchers, clinicians, and patients will be essential for advancing our understanding of this complex condition and improving the quality of life for those affected.

Acknowledgements

We would like to express our sincere gratitude to Veysel Barış Turhan and Bahadır Kartal for their invaluable support and contributions to this work. Their expertize and assistance have been instrumental in the completion of this chapter. Thank you for your unwavering support and encouragement.

The author acknowledges the use of ChatGPT for language polishing of the manuscript.

Conflict of interest

The authors declare no conflict of interest.

Author details

Merve Konal
Department of Obstetrics and Gynecology, Gynecologic Oncology Department, Hitit University Erol Olçok Training and Research Hospital, Çorum, Turkey

*Address all correspondence to: mervekonal@gmail.com

References

[1] Zondervan KT, Becker CM, Missmer SA. Endometriosis. The New England Journal of Medicine. 2020;**382**:1244-1256

[2] Simoens S, Hummelshoj L, D'Hooghe T. Endometriosis: Cost estimates and methodological perspective. Human Reproduction Update. 2007;**13**:395-404

[3] Prescott J, Farland LV, Tobias DK, Gaskins AJ, Spiegelman D, Chavarro JE, et al. A prospective cohort study of endometriosis and subsequent risk of infertility. Human Reproduction. 2016;**31**:1475-1482

[4] Ghiasi M, Kulkarni MT, Missmer SA. Is endometriosis more common and more severe than it was 30 years ago? Journal of Minimally Invasive Gynecology. 2020;**27**:452-461

[5] Saunders PTK, Horne AW. Endometriosis: Etiology, pathobiology, and therapeutic prospects. Cell. 2021;**184**:2807-2824

[6] Missmer SA, Cramer DW. The epidemiology of endometriosis. Obstetrics and Gynecology Clinics of North America. 2003;**30**:1-19, vii

[7] Bian Y, Yuan L, Yang X, Weng L, Zhang Y, Bai H, et al. SMURF1-mediated ubiquitylation of SHP-1 promotes cell proliferation and invasion of endometrial stromal cells in endometriosis. Annals of Translational Medicine. 2021;**9**:362

[8] Ahn SH, Singh V, Tayade C. Biomarkers in endometriosis: Challenges and opportunities. Fertility and Sterility. 2017;**107**:523-532

[9] Young VJ, Brown JK, Saunders PT, Horne AW. The role of the peritoneum in the pathogenesis of endometriosis. Human Reproduction Update. 2013;**19**:558-569

[10] Kuznetsov L, Dworzynski K, Davies M, Overton C, Guideline Committee. Diagnosis and management of endometriosis: Summary of NICE guidance. BMJ. 2017;**358**:j3935

[11] Brown J, Pan A, Hart RJ. Gonadotrophin-releasing hormone analogues for pain associated with endometriosis. Cochrane Database of Systematic Reviews. 2010;**2010**:CD008475

[12] Donnez J, Taylor HS, Taylor RN, Akin MD, Tatarchuk TF, Wilk K, et al. Treatment of endometriosis-associated pain with linzagolix, an oral gonadotropin-releasing hormone-antagonist: A randomized clinical trial. Fertility and Sterility. 2020;**114**:44-55

[13] Brown J, Kives S, Akhtar M. Progestagens and anti-progestagens for pain associated with endometriosis. Cochrane Database of Systematic Reviews. 2012;**2012**:CD002122

[14] Wu D, Hu M, Hong L, Hong S, Ding W, Min J, et al. Clinical efficacy of add-back therapy in treatment of endometriosis: A meta-analysis. Archives of Gynecology and Obstetrics. 2014;**290**:513-523

[15] Carlyle D, Khader T, Lam D, Vadivelu N, Shiwlochan D. Endometriosis pain management: A review. Current Pain and Headache Reports. 2020;**24**:1-9

[16] Tassinari V, Smeriglio A, Stillittano V, Trombetta D, Zilli R, Tassinari R, et al. Endometriosis treatment: Role of natural

polyphenols as anti-inflammatory agents. Nutrients. 2023;**15**(13):2967

[17] Guan Q, Velho RV, Sehouli J, Mechsner S. Endometriosis and opioid receptors: Are opioids a possible/promising treatment for endometriosis? International Journal of Molecular Sciences. 2023;**24**(2):1633

[18] Adamietz A, Boosz A, Mueller A, Hornung D, Trunk K, Beckmann MW, et al. Complementary and alternative medicine (CAM) in women with endometriosis. European Journal of Obstetrics, Gynecology, and Reproductive Biology. 2021;**262**:7-12

[19] Singh SS, Gude K, Perdeaux E, Gattrell WT, Becker CM. Surgical outcomes in patients with endometriosis: A systematic review. Journal of Obstetrics and Gynaecology Canada. 2020;**42**(7):881-888

[20] Malvezzi H, Marengo EB, Podgaec S, Piccinato CDA. Endometriosis: Current challenges in modeling a multifactorial disease of unknown etiology. Journal of Translational Medicine. 2020;**18**:1-21

[21] Mei C, Gong W, Wang X, Lv Y, Zhang Y, Wu S, et al. Anti-angiogenic therapy in ovarian cancer: Current understandings and prospects of precision medicine. Frontiers in Pharmacology. 2023;**14**:1147717

[22] Clemenza S, Vannuccini S, Ruotolo A, Capezzuoli T, Petraglia F. Advances in targeting estrogen synthesis and receptors in patients with endometriosis. Expert Opinion on Investigational Drugs. 2022;**31**(11):1227-1238

[23] Abokhrais IM, Denison FC, Whitaker LHR, Saunders PTK, Doust A, Williams LJ, et al. A two-arm parallel double-blind randomised controlled pilot trial of the efficacy of Omega-3 polyunsaturated fatty acids for the treatment of women with endometriosis-associated pain (PurFECT1). PLoS ONE. 2020;**15**:e0227695

[24] Loving S, Nordling J, Jaszczak P, Thomsen T. Does evidence support physiotherapy management of adult female chronic pelvic pain? A systematic review. Scandinavian Journal of Pain. 2012;**3**:70-81

[25] Cohen SP, Vase L, Hooten WM. Chronic pain: An update on burden, best practices, and new advances. Lancet. 2021;**397**:2082-2097

[26] Williams ACC, Fisher E, Hearn L, Eccleston C. Psychological therapies for the management of chronic pain (excluding headache) in adults. Cochrane Database of Systematic Reviews. 2020;**8**:CD007407

[27] Guo SW. Recurrence of endometriosis and its control. Human Reproduction Update. 2009;**15**:441-461

[28] Salliss ME, Farland LV, Mahnert ND, Herbst-Kralovetz MM. The role of gut and genital microbiota and the estrobolome in endometriosis, infertility and chronic pelvic pain. Human Reproduction Update. 2021;**28**:92-131

Chapter 4

Pain Management for Women with Endometriosis

Daniela Rangel-Santos, German William Rangel and Sudhir Diwan

Abstract

Endometriosis is a leading cause of chronic pelvic pain in women and requires multidimensional lifelong management strategies. This chapter comprehensively reviews the multidisciplinary approaches to pain management in women with endometriosis, emphasizing both pharmacological and interventional strategies. Medical management includes non-steroidal anti-inflammatory drugs (NSAIDs) and hormonal contraceptives as the first line of treatment, providing adequate pain relief for many patients. Other pharmacological options include tricyclic and serotonin and norepinephrine reuptake inhibitors (SNRI) antidepressants, calcium channel blockers, GnRH agonists/antagonists, and aromatase inhibitors. Some disadvantages related to pharmacological treatment include inhibition of ovulation, side effects of medications, and high recurrence of pain after discontinuation of treatment. Surgical management is usually delayed due to the risk of pelvic organ damage and postoperative adhesion formation. Physical and behavioral therapy are encouraged as a comprehensive approach to chronic pelvic pain. Interventional pain management techniques have emerged as a therapeutic option providing adequate pain control without impairing fertility. Neuromodulatory techniques such as peripheral nerve stimulation, dorsal root ganglion, and spinal cord stimulation could be a promising line of treatment for patients with refractory pain.

Keywords: chronic pelvic pain, endometriosis, percutaneous neuromodulation therapies, peripheral nerve stimulation, dorsal root ganglion stimulation, spinal cord stimulation

1. Introduction

Endometriosis is a chronic debilitating disease characterized by the formation of endometrial-like tissue outside of the uterine cavity [1, 2]. It affects approximately 10% of reproductive-aged women around the world and it is present in 20–50% of women struggling with infertility and 71–87% of women suffering from chronic pelvic pain [1, 3]. The most common ectopic locations of endometrial glands and stroma are the pelvic peritoneum, the ovaries, and the rectovaginal septum [4].

Unlike eutopic endometrium, endometriosis lesions often contain blood, cysts, and fibrous tissue [5]. It has been proposed that endometriosis is an estrogen-dependent condition and that this aberrant tissue responds to hormonal stimulation and undergoes cyclical growth and shedding [6].

Pain is described as the most debilitating symptom of endometriosis and is usually one of the most challenging symptoms to manage given the presence of both somatic and visceral pain [7]. Presentation of pain most frequently includes dysmenorrhea, cyclic and acyclic pelvic pain, dyspareunia, dyschezia in patients with bowel involvement, dysuria in patients with bladder involvement, and radiating lower back pain [8]. Other nonspecific symptoms include headaches, dizziness, and chronic fatigue. As a result, endometriosis impacts the physical, mental, emotional, and social spheres of life for many women [6].

The precise etiopathogenesis of endometriosis is unclear, involving multiple processes and a combination of genetic and epigenetic factors [9]. There has been described three distinct forms of endometriosis: superficial or peritoneal endometriosis (endometriotic implants on the surface of pelvic peritoneum and ovaries), ovarian endometriomas (ovarian cysts lined by endometrioid mucosa), and deep infiltrative or rectovaginal endometriotic nodules (a solid mass comprising endometriotic tissue mixed with adipose and fibromuscular tissue in the space between the vagina and the rectum) [10]. Recently, nerve entrapment by endometriosis has been proposed as a fourth form of clinical presentation [11].

2. Pathogenesis of pain

Pain secondary to endometriosis has been associated with both inflammatory and neuropathic components that contribute to the severity of symptoms. The International Association for the Study of Pain (IASP) defines neuropathic pain as pain that arises as a direct consequence of a lesion or disease affecting the somatosensory system [12]. It has been proposed that endometriotic lesions growing in the peritoneal cavity stimulate the production of proinflammatory cytokines and growth factors. The resulting inflammation could lead to peripheral nerve sensitization associated with neuropathic pain [13]. The peritoneal fluid of women with endometriosis has shown an increased level of inflammatory cytokines (e.g. IL-1, IL-6, IL-8), leptin, and TNF-α [14–16]. Additionally, the expression of peroxisome proliferator-activated receptor-γ (PPAR-γ) has been correlated with clinical presentation of dysmenorrhea and dyspareunia. Contrarily, treatment regimens that reduce IL-8, PAPP-A, midkin, and progestogen-associated endometrial protein have demonstrated a reduction in pain presentation [17]. Endometriotic lesions usually present a higher nerve density and expression of nerve growth factor, commonly leading to the development of chronic neuropathic pain [18]. It has also been proposed that inflammatory changes interact with the central nervous system leading to chronic pain. In accordance with this theory, structural changes in regional gray matter in women with endometriosis have been found [19, 20]. Moreover, it has been proposed that endometriotic lesions may infiltrate adjacent nerve fibers as they grow, leading to hyperalgesia. Recent studies have linked nerve fiber proximity to increased pain and indicate that pain generation is directly related to the location of the ectopic endometriotic tissue and the involvement of the peripheral nervous system in that region [21]. Therefore, an effective treatment requires a deep understanding of the mechanisms generating pain and a multidisciplinary treatment approach [9].

Endometriosis can also result in neurological symptoms when the central or peripheral nervous system is affected, manifesting as cyclic radiculopathy of the lower limbs, groin and buttocks, leg pain, pelvic pain, and in more severe cases even urinary incontinence and paraplegia [9]. Physical findings that may be present include analgesic gait, gluteal atrophy, groin pain, ankle dorsiflexion weakness, and worsening of pain with hip movement. Abdominal wall endometriosis can appear between 3 months to 10 years after abdominal surgery, presenting as incisional endometriosis at the anterior abdominal wall and often mistaken for other conditions (e.g. hernias, abscesses, granulomas, lipomas) [22]. Endometriosis affecting the sacral plexus is rare and can cause sciatic pain, hip pain, anal pain, pudendal pain, and gluteal atrophy secondary to superior and inferior gluteal nerve involvement [23]. Neuropathic pain is often described as a burning, electrical, and cramping sensation in the compromised region, such as the hypogastrium, perineum, vaginal opening, or anus [24]. **Table 1** summarizes the main types of mechanisms of pain related to endometriosis according to the structures involved.

2.1 Relevant neuroanatomy

A complete medical history and a thorough physical examination are necessary to differentiate between various pain generators properly. Pain related to endometriosis may include a visceral origin from pelvic organs (defined as persistent or recurrent pain that originates from internal organs of the abdominal and pelvic cavities), somatic origin due to muscle and ligament involvement, and neuropathic characteristics in case of nerve infiltration [12]. A clear understanding of pelvic innervation is crucial when stablishing an interventional pain management target.

Mechanism of pain
Endometrial cells that have grown outside the uterus can directly invade or irritate peripheral nerves, impacting the nerve fibers in the pelvic region.
Peripheral and central sensitization.
Scar tissue formation by pressing or pulling on nerves.
Nonspecific bowel and bladder symptoms.
Compression or irritation of the sciatic nerve.
Stretching of the sacral hypogastric fascia.
Pudendal neuropathy (S2, S3, S4).
Involvement of the superior gluteal nerve (L4, S5, S1).
Involvement of the inferior gluteal nerve.
Involvement of the cluneal nerves.
Involvement of posterior femoral cutaneous nerve.
Root nerve involvement.
Abdominal wall nerve entrapment.
Inguinal nerve entrapment.
Trigger points in the iliococcygeus, pubococcygeus, and puborectalis muscles.
Sacral network involvement.

Table 1.
Mechanisms of pain generation in endometriosis.

Afferent sensory roots emerge from the dorsal horn of the spinal cord and travel to the periphery until they collect in a bundle of pseudo-unipolar cell bodies named the dorsal root ganglion (DRG) [25]. Efferent motor roots emerge from the ventral horn of the spinal cord and converge with the dorsal roots to form mixed spinal nerves. As each spinal nerve travels peripherally, it divides into the dorsal and ventral primary rami and forms the peripheral nerves [26].

The ilioinguinal and iliohypogastric nerves (L1), the genitofemoral nerve (L1–L2), and the pudendal nerves (S2, S3, S4) transmit somatic sensory and motor innervation of the pelvis. The pudendal nerves supply mixed innervation to the perineum, the external genital, and the anal region. Visceral or autonomic innervation goes through the sympathetic and parasympathetic systems, with sympathetic trunk fibers having their cell bodies in the thoracolumbar DRG and parasympathetic trunk fibers having their cell bodies in the sacral DRG [26]. The superior hypogastric plexus, inferior hypogastric plexus, the splanchnic nerves, and the impar ganglion carry the sympathetic innervation of the pelvis.

The DRG has gained protagonism in recent years, since now evidence supports its role in neuropathic pain modulation. Previously considered a passive structure that merely connected the central and peripheral nervous systems, it has been shown that stimulation of DRG decreases neuron hyperexcitability secondary to afferent nerve injury [25].

3. Pain management

There is no substantial evidence to determine the superiority of surgical vs. medical management of pain symptoms. A systematic review of 23 studies and 1847 patients reported no statistically significant pain improvement after undergoing surgical treatment compared to medical treatment modalities [27, 28]. Providers are encouraged to consider all modalities, suggesting medical management as the first line of treatment, but understanding that the combination of medical and surgical treatments amounts to the highest success rate [29].

3.1 Surgical management

The surgical approach ranges from excision and/or ablation of the endometriotic lesions to hysterectomy with or without oophorectomy. Ablation of lesions can be performed using monopolar or bipolar cautery, laser, or argon gas. Excision of deeply infiltrating lesions is recommended, and medical therapy following surgical treatment provides a longer symptomatic relief [27]. Furthermore, it has been reported that patients with moderate disease experience a higher improvement of pain symptoms than those with mild or minimal disease. Recurrence of pain occurs in 20–40% of patients who undergo surgical treatment. However, multiple surgical procedures should be avoided due to the risk of adhesions, secondary pelvic pain, and decreased ovarian reserve [30]. Regarding ovarian endometriomas, medical treatment may lead to a temporary reduction of cyst size but has not shown complete resolution of the lesions [31]. Surgery should be the primary option of treatment for large or symptomatic endometriomas. Cyst removal has proven a greater improvement in dysmenorrhea, dyspareunia, and pelvic pain. Simple drainage, fenestration, or ablation of the cyst wall is associated with 80–100% recurrence at 6 months and is not recommended as final treatment [32].

Other ablative techniques are less utilized due to unsatisfactory pain resolution, technical difficulty, and related adverse effects [33]. Laparoscopic uterosacral nerve ablation or resection targets the efferent fibers within the uterosacral ligaments to disrupt the primary innervation of the cervical sensory fibers. While the rate of complications is low, uterine prolapse and ureter transection have been reported [34]. Presacral neurectomy consists of incising the superior hypogastric nerve plexus 1 cm caudal to the aortic bifurcation. Because of the plexus' location near the venous plexus and major vessels, this procedure is technically challenging and carries a significant risk of bleeding and postoperative complications that include urinary retention and constipation [35]. The rates of recurrent pain were similar to those who underwent conservative surgery, seemingly offering no further benefit over the traditional laparoscopic approach [33].

Regarding hysterectomy with bilateral salpingo-oophorectomy, it should be only considered in patients with advanced and treatment-resistant endometriosis who are satisfied with parity. Debulking of disease and associated menopause leads to atrophy of endometriosis tissue with a lower recurrence of symptoms [27, 36]. The decision to perform salpingo-oophorectomy should consider early menopause and the need for hormone replacement therapy [36].

3.2 Medical management

Medical management for endometriosis includes NSAIDs, oral contraceptives, progestogens, danazol, GnRH-agonists, and anti-progestogens [37]. **Table 2** indicates the recommended treatment regimen for each drug group as stated by the American Academy of Family Physicians [3].

3.2.1 NSAIDS

NSAIDs are commonly employed as the first line of treatment due to availability and manageable side effects. NSAID*s* inhibit prostaglandin production that contributes to inflammation and pain. Anti-prostaglandin agents are effective in the treatment of primary dysmenorrhea, but their effectiveness for endometriosis pain is yet to be established [38, 39]. A 2015 Cochrane review compared NSAIDs to placebo and no recommendation could be established. Even though pain scores were lower for the NSAIDs group, evidence was inconclusive regarding quantifiable data such as quality of life or effect on daily activities [38]. These findings were supported by a more recent 2017 Cochrane review where only two randomized controlled trials (RCT) comparing NSAIDs versus placebo for endometriosis-related pain were found [40, 41]. Results showed a difference between NSAIDs and placebo for overall pain relief, however, unintended effects of treatment or requirement for additional medication remained unclear. No data was provided on other secondary outcomes such as quality of life, the effects on daily activities, work and school absenteeism, the number of women requiring more invasive treatment, and patient's satisfaction with treatment. Additionally, no evidence supports whether an individual NSAID is more effective than another [42]. Both reviews suggested that patients should be informed of secondary effects that could be caused by NSAIDs prior to their prescription [38, 42]. Larger and more recent randomized control trials are needed to update these results.

3.2.2 Neuroleptics

Pelvic pain secondary to endometriosis has been found to encompass a multifaceted neural mechanism that includes nociceptive as well as neuropathic pathways.

Medication	Indication	Dosing
Depot MDA (Depo-Provera)	Pain relief	150 mg intramuscularly every 3 months
MDPA (Provera)	Pain relief	30 to 100 mg daily (orally)
Combined OCPs	Pain relief	0.02 to 0.03 mg ethinyl estradiol and 0.15 mg desogestrel daily for 6 months
Levonorgestrel intrauterine system (Mirena)	Pain relief after surgery	Intrauterine system
Gonadotropin-releasing hormone analogues: • Goserelin (Zoladex) • Leuprolide (Lupron) • Triptorelin (Trelstar Depot)	Pain relief	3.75 mg of leuprolide injected every four weeks or 3.6 mg of goserelin implanted subcutaneously for 6 months
Nafarelin (Synarel)	Pain relief	200 mcg intranasally twice daily for 6 months
Danazol (Danocrine)	Pain relief	200 mg given orally three times daily; 400 mg given orally twice daily for 6 months
Gestrinone	Pain relief	2.5 mg orally twice a week for 6 months

MDPA = medroxyprogesterone acetate; OCPs = oral contraceptive pills (Adapted from Gharaei et Gholampoor).

Table 2.
Medical treatment for endometriosis pain.

For patients who present with significant nerve damage from endometriosis, persistent pain may follow despite excision of the disease, and severity of the disease may not correlate with reported pain. Pregabalin, gabapentin, and calcium channel blockers could be a therapeutic option for these patients by decreasing glutamine uptake, norepinephrine, and substance P and stabilizing central and peripheral membranes. These drugs are conventionally used for neuropathic pain but also for nonspecific pain conditions [43, 44].

Tricyclic antidepressants are another first-line treatment for many neuropathic chronic pain conditions, by increasing available norepinephrine that inhibits descending pain pathways [44]. An RCT in women with chronic pelvic pain comparing the use of amitriptyline, gabapentin, and amitriptyline/gabapentin combined for 24 months reported significantly reduced pain in each group and showed fewer side effects in the gabapentin group [45].

Almeida et al. conducted a systematic review to evaluate the effect of neuromodulatory drugs on the intensity of chronic pelvic pain in women [46]. Among the seven studies included, four showed improvement in pain with the use of neuromodulator drugs for chronic pelvic pain. However, the most powerful and high-quality study did not show pain improvement. Additionally, no studies specifically evaluating pain in women with endometriosis were found. There is still no high-quality evidence to either indicate or avoid the use of neuromodulatory drugs in endometriosis, and further high-quality studies, especially randomized controlled trials, are needed to support the use of these drugs in the treatment of women with endometriosis.

3.2.3 Combined oral contraceptives

The utilization of combined oral contraceptives inhibits the production of gonadal estrogen by suppressing ovarian activity through a negative feedback axis.

Consequently, the release of estrogen-induced release of prostaglandins is reduced and inflammation decreases [47]. In addition, combined hormonal drugs are thought to cause decidualization followed by atrophy of endometrial tissue [48, 49]. When administered for endometriosis, combined hormonal contraceptives should be used continuously in comparison to cyclic administration for symptom control [50].

3.2.4 Progesterones

Norethindrone acetate, depot medroxyprogesterone acetate (MPA), levonorgestrel-releasing intrauterine system (LNG-IUS), and dienogest are some of the most frequently used progestogens in women with endometriosis. Progestogens are proposed to work through several mechanisms [49]:

1. decidualization and consequent endometrial atrophy.

2. progestogen-induced suppression of matrix metalloproteinases, enzymes that influence the growth and ectopic implantation of endometrium.

3. Inhibition of angiogenesis.

Treatment with MPA, dydrogesterone, or norethindrone acetate has been shown to reduce pain scores by 70–100% [1]. MPA has proven to be an effective treatment with combined oral contraceptives, danazol, and GnRH-agonists. Dienogest was reported as significantly better than placebo and as effective as GnRH-agonists with a more favorable side effect profile [51]. Levonorgestrel-releasing intrauterine systems have been proven more effective in reducing dysmenorrhea after laparoscopic surgery when compared to expectant management and have been associated with a significant decrease in the extension of lesions encountered during second-look laparoscopy 6 months later [52].

3.2.5 Gonadotropin-releasing hormone agonists

GnRH agonist analogues have been studied more extensively than other medical lines of treatment [27, 37]. Modified analogues present a longer half-life and bind to the receptors in the pituitary gland, interrupting the pulsatile stimulation of endogenous GnRH [53]. Consequently, downregulation of the pituitary-ovarian axis and hypoestrogenism induce amenorrhea and progressive atrophy of endometrial tissue [49]. Drug presentations include nafarelin acetate calibrated nasal spray, short-acting formulation for daily injection, and depot formulation every *1–3 months* in the form of leuprolide acetate or goserelin acetate [29]. The main side effects reported are related to the induced hypoestrogenic state: hot flushes, vaginal dryness, decreased libido, mood swings, headache, and bone mineral depletion [54].

A Cochrane review demonstrated GnRH-analogues to be more effective for pain than placebo and similarly effective to LNG-IUS and danazol, with one long-term follow-up demonstrating a 53% reduction in recurrence of symptoms at 24 months after six-month treatment with GnRH-agonists [55]. Combined therapy with norethindrone acetate or an estrogen-progestogen regimen has been proposed as an alternative to reduce estrogen deprivation effects and should be started at the same time of GnRH [27]. It has been proposed that the amount of estrogen/progesterone necessary to prevent hypoestrogenism symptoms is less than that which would stimulate endometriotic tissue formation [56].

3.2.6 Gonadotropin-releasing hormone antagonists

GnRH antagonists, such as Elagolix, suppress the gonadotropin hormone production from the pituitary gland and cause a dose-dependent hypoestrogenic state. In contrast to GnRH agonists, they avoid the initial surge in LH and GSH and provide an immediate effect [57]. Side effects may include symptoms of hypoestrogenism such as hot flashes, headaches, insomnia, and higher lipid levels. Elagolix has been recently approved in the USA for moderate to severe pain related to endometriosis, and its studies have shown a significant short-term reduction of dysmenorrhea and non-menstrual pelvic pain with adequate maintenance of response [58, 59].

3.2.7 Danazol

Danazol is a 17 alpha-ethinyltestosterone derivative that inhibits the LH peak and steroidogenesis through the increase of free testosterone levels [49]. Its effectivity for the treatment of endometriosis-related pain has proven to be superior to placebo and comparable to GnRH-agonists [60]. Side effects include hirsutism, acne, weight gain, and deepening of voice. Danazol can be administered orally and through vaginal or intrauterine delivery systems [37].

3.2.8 Experimental treatments: Gestrinone

Ethylnorgestrienone is an antiprogestational steroid that produces a progesterone withdrawal effect at the endometrial cellular level and inhibits ovarian steroidogenesis. It is administered orally from 2.5 to 10 mg daily to weekly basis, showing an effectiveness comparable to danazol and GnRH-agonists [55]. Side effects are associated with its androgenic and anti-estrogenic effects [49]. Gestrinone is not approved for use in the USA, but its use is currently approved for Europe.

3.2.9 Experimental treatments: Aromatase inhibitors

Aromatase inhibitors are still under current investigation, with low-impact studies showing effectiveness in endometriosis-related pelvic pain treatment for women pre- and postmenopause [61]. Endometriotic tissue exhibits a higher level of aromatase activity in comparison to eutopic endometrium. This results in an increase of local estrogen and favors endometriosis formation, explaining the persistence of endometriotic tissue in postmenopausal women and in those patients receiving treatment with GnRH agonists [27]. In women who have not undergone menopause, aromatase inhibitors should be used in combination with an additional agent that down-regulates the ovaries and protects bone density such as progestogens, combined oral contraceptives, or GnRH [62].

3.3 Interventional pain management treatments

Endometriosis-related pain could be treated effectively using interventional pain management strategies. It has been stated that refractory pain due to endometriosis should respond to nerve blocks depending on the site of involvement [63]. The sympathetic nervous system plays an essential role in the transmission of pain from internal organs, independently of its cause [9]. The superior hypogastric plexus block (SHPB) is one commonly used approach in treating persistent pelvic and rectal pain that does not respond to conservative treatment [64, 65]. Located ventrally to the abdominal aorta, the superior hypogastric plexus innervates hindgut structures like the descendent and sigmoid colon, the proximal rectum, and pelvic organs such as the uterus and ovaries [66]. The SHPB procedure can be performed through either a paravertebral or transdiscal approach and has been reported to significantly improve the quality of life and mental health status of women with endometriosis [67]. The choice of analgesic injectate should be carefully done by the physician considering the maximum analgesic effect while minimizing the side effects experienced by patients. Typical agents used include steroids, bupivacaine, and chemical agents such as (5–10%) and ethanol (50–100%) [68]. The inferior hypogastric plexus block (IHPB) is a less popular technique for the treatment of pelvic, perineal, and genital pain due to its challenging location in the presacral space that conditions a higher risk of nerve damage, vascular puncture, rectal lesion, presacral hematoma, and infection [69].

The ganglion impar block is another useful technique for the treatment of malignant vulvar, rectal, and anal pain; intractable sacral and perineal pain and coccydynia [70]. Other techniques for treating endometriosis-associated pain include performing S3 pulsed radiofrequency in combination with IHPB or botulinum toxin injection and myofascial pain trigger points [71, 72].

Targeting the sympathetic axes has been shown to be useful in controlling visceral pelvic pain. The technique of choice should be based on clinical presentation and the structures that are compromised [73]. SHPB is most effective for pain involving pelvic viscera (e.g. uterus, ovaries, and bladder), the rectum, and hindgut structures [70]. When treating perineal, genital, presacral, and low pelvic pain, an IHPB is most recommended [74, 75]. Ganglion impar block is an option in cases with involvement of the vulva and anal orifice, presence of intractable sacral and/or perineal pain, or coccydynia. Gharaei and Gholampoor proposed an approach to the choice of interventional technique based on location and clinical presentation which is represented in **Figure 1** [9].

3.3.1 Hydrodissection with dextrose for peripheral nerve entrapment

Peripheral nerve entrapment is an underrecognized entity when treating patients with endometriosis and results in the persistence of pain and disability despite the treatment offered. Entrapment of the nerve occurs due to anatomical or pathological structures that cause increased pressure and lead to several mechanisms of nerve damage, producing a segmental injury of the nerve. Symptoms can range from mild discomfort and numbness to debilitating pain and even paralysis. Injury of the nerve is produced by mechanical compression, contraction, and excessive stretching that leads to chronic hypoxia and inflammation. The resulting pain is of neuropathic characteristic which patients may describe as a numbing, tingling, burning, shooting, lancinating, or electric shock sensation [76]. Since central sensibilization can increase pain over time, it is important to perform an early intervention. Hydrodissection consists of a deep perineural injection into the compressing tissue or fascia, releasing the trapped nerves while diluting and washing away the local inflammatory response [77]. Nerve structures are identified under ultrasound and a perineural injection with 5% dextrose is administered. Dextrose reduces neuropathic inflammation and dissects the endometrial tissues. It has been proposed that dextrose delivered to the perineurial soft tissues may aid in nerve recovery by reducing adhesion and damage from chronic contraction and enhancing blood flow [78].

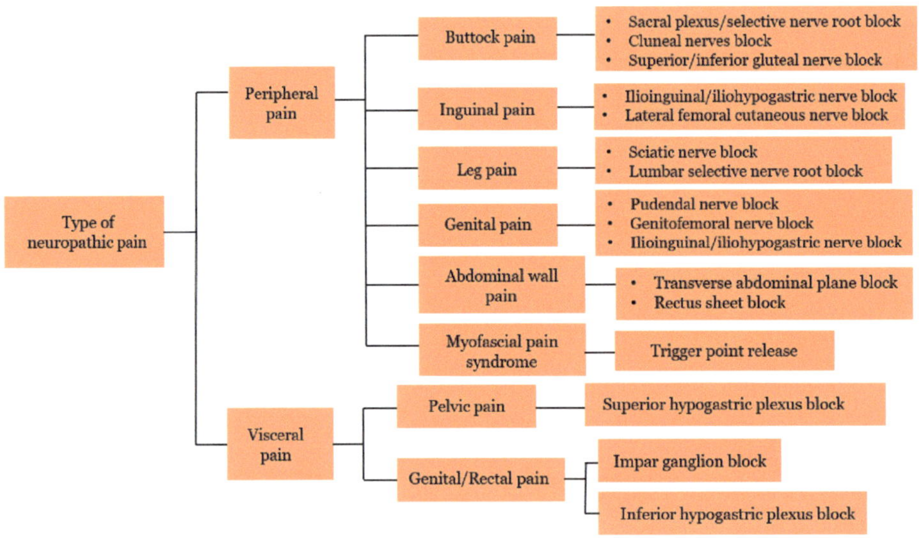

Figure 1.
Algorithmic approach to interventional pain management for neuropathic pain in endometriosis (Adapted from Gharaei et al.).

3.4 Advanced neuromodulation techniques

Neuromodulation consists of electrical stimulation or administration of pharmacological agents that alter and moderate pain signals. Neuromodulation use has been described for the treatment of chronic pelvic pain, including spinal cord stimulation (SCS), dorsal root ganglion (DRG) stimulation, sacral nerve roots stimulation, and peripheral nerve stimulation (PNS) [79].

3.4.1 Spinal cord stimulator

SCS has been proposed as a therapeutical option for refractory pelvic pain and could be effective in endometriosis-related pain management [80]. Case series and prospective studies have been developed with variations in lead placement. Kapural et al. reported the first case series of SCS for refractory visceral pelvic pain in six women using an anterograde approach with lead placement at T11-T12. A significant reduction in the mean visual analog scale (VAS) score was reported, as well as a reduction in pain disability index and opioid use in morphine milligram equivalents (MME) [81]. Buffenior et al. conducted a prospective study evaluating the role of SCS of the conus medullaris applied to 27 patients with refractory pudendal neuralgia. A total of 20 patients had a positive response during the trial period and underwent permanent electrode implantation, remaining long-term responders. At 15-month follow-up, the mean estimated percent improvement (EPI) was 55.5% [82]. A case series conducted by Simopoulous et al. followed three patients who underwent implantation of a high-frequency 10 KHz SCS mediated at the conus medullaris for different clinical presentations of refractory neuropathic pelvic pain, reporting satisfactory pain relief for all patients at long-term follow-up [83]. A prospective, multicenter trial performed by Tate et al. evaluated the efficacy of 10-KHz SCS in patients with chronic pelvic pain. Among the 21 patients who underwent the trial, 17 were positive respondents and 14 of them received a permanent SCS implantation. A total of 77% of the patients who underwent implantation reported pain relief over 50% and the mean VAS score decreased by 72% [84]. Hunter et al. described lead placement at higher thoracic levels for the management of chronic pelvic pain, with four patients who received SCS lead placement in the mid-thoracic region, two patients with T6 level lead placement, and two patients who underwent T7 level trial. A total of three patients in the series had a positive trial response and received permanent implantation [85]. A prospective chart review completed by De Andres et al. found limited effectiveness of retrograde neurostimulation in the treatment of perineal pain, describing technical limitations and the complex pelvic innervation that does not subscribe to a specific dermatome [86].

3.4.2 Dorsal root ganglion stimulation

Schu et al. reviewed the use of DRG stimulation in patients with groin pain. A total of 29 patients were included and taken to trial with stimulation of the DRG between T12 and L4, resulting in 25 patients who were respondent and eligible for implantation. Among the implanted patients, 82.6% experienced a reduction in pain superior to 50%. These results could indicate that neuromodulation of the DRG is effective in treating pelvic neuropathic pain syndromes, including endometriosis [87]. Hunter et al. conducted the first case series of DRG stimulation in patients with chronic pelvic pain that had not responded to conservative treatment and other interventional pain management techniques. A total of seven patients were trialed successfully and underwent DRG stimulator implants with lead placement over L1 and S2 DRGs bilaterally. Pain relief report was satisfactory at follow-up, opioid consumption decreased, and some of the patients additionally reported improvement in urination and sexual function. The authors proposed that the lead placement generated an upstream and downstream effect through crosstalk between the DRG and the ganglia, and suggested L1 as the most cephalad level in which inferior pain signals get transmitted to the brain. Stimulation of the L1 DRG stops the upper lumbar plexus signaling to the brain and S2 DRG stimulation interrupts pain signals originating from the lower lumbar and sacral plexus [88].

3.4.3 Peripheral nerve stimulation

The main targets for PNS described for chronic pelvic pain include the sacral, pudendal, posterior tibial, genitofemoral, ilioinguinal, and iliohypogastric nerves according to pain localization. PNS leads are aimed to be placed parallel to the peripheral nerve. Among sacral nerves, the most common target is the S3 root. Siegel et al. and Paszkiewicz et al. studied the effectiveness of sacral nerve stimulation in intractable pelvic pain, performing a successful trial in 10 patients with lead placement in S3 or S4 foramen. At a median follow-up time of 19 months, the mean reduction of VAS was superior to 50% [89]. Martelucci et al. included 27 patients with chronic pelvic pain in their study, of which 15 were trialed successfully and underwent implantation, finding sustained pain relief at 60 months follow-up. Additionally, positive response to calcium channel blockers such as pregabalin and gabapentin was found to be a predictor of positive response to sacral neuromodulation, while poorly localized pain was an indicator of poor response [90]. Vancaillie et al. conducted one of the largest studies involving PNS consisting of a case series of 52 patients evaluating sacral neuromodulation for pelvic pain, with promising results indicating that sacral neuromodulation could represent an effective treatment for intractable chronic pelvic pain [91].

Further high-quality research is needed to provide a strong recommendation for the use of advanced neuromodulation techniques in endometriosis-related pain and stablish a consensus on neuromodulatory targets. Decisions on what technique is most convenient should be based on pain location and a thorough medical evaluation. Possible risks and complications, patient's expectations, and the implications of a medical device implantation should be discussed prior to the procedure.

3.5 Adjuvant therapies

3.5.1 Exercise

Physical exercise has been considered an adjuvant treatment for dysmenorrhea for decades, considering that exercise releases anti-inflammatory cytokines and reduces cortisol levels, leading to a reduction in prostaglandin release [92]. Additionally, the skeletal muscle is believed to act as an endocrine organ, releasing myokines with muscular contraction. These myokines are theorized to exert direct effects on the muscle and other distal organs such as the liver, pancreas, and adipose tissue [93]. Carroquino-Garcia et al. concluded in their systematic review that therapeutic exercise for a period of 8 to 12 weeks reduces pain intensity and duration of dysmenorrhea [94]. A recent systematic review by Mira et al. reported an improvement in pain and quality of life when an exercise protocol was added to different pharmacological interventions, however, due to the sample size of individual studies, the evidence was not considered significant [95]. Given the low risk of the intervention and the potential benefits to the patients' overall health, exercise in conjunction with other treatment modalities could be encouraged to alleviate symptoms [96].

3.5.2 Acupuncture

Studies regarding the use of acupuncture in endometriosis-related pain are increasing worldwide. Two randomized trials evaluated specific acupuncture compared to sham acupuncture for endometriosis-related pain finding significantly better pain control with real acupuncture [97, 98]. Xu et al. demonstrated in their systematic review that acupuncture had a beneficial effect on pain reduction compared to other treatments such as traditional Chinese medicine, medication, or placebo [99]. Acupuncture has been suggested to activate peripheral analgesic mechanisms such as the release of endogenous opioids and to participate in the modulation of several anti-inflammatory pathways, and inhibitory control mechanisms [100]. These findings were corroborated by a recent meta-analysis involving the use of acupuncture compared to placebo for women with endometriosis-related pelvic pain [95].

3.5.3 Behavioral health

Chronic pelvic pain has been associated with a higher prevalence of psychologic symptoms such as depression and anxiety, and a significant reduction in work productivity [101]. Most women with endometriosis and pelvic pain present some level of impairment in their mental health and quality of life associated to the chronicity and emotional aspects of the disease [102]. Furthermore, around 67% of women with endometriosis experience problems in the relationship with their partners, mainly due to painful intercourse [103, 104]. This complex interplay of factors, also referred to as the biopsychosocial injuries caused by the disease, could induce a vicious cycle that compromises the base treatment, whether it is pharmacological or surgical [105]. Buggio et al. described a series of interventions for women with endometriosis, including psychotherapy and sexual therapy, that approach the self-management of physical, psychological, and sexual symptoms obtaining positive outcomes when integrated into the clinical treatment of pain [106]. Practitioners should consider referral to a mental health professional early in the treatment to address the psychological and social factors that contribute to pain.

3.5.4 Pelvic floor physical therapy

Chronic pelvic pain leads to muscle contraction and postural changes that exacerbate musculoskeletal pain. Physical therapy, including heat therapy, has been proposed to enhance the relaxation of abdominal muscles and increase pelvic blood circulation [92]. There is no strong evidence with a well-described methodology for recommending the different forms of physiotherapy that may be most effective in the treatment of endometriosis. Current reviews indicate that transcutaneous electrical nerve stimulation (TENS), pulsed high-intensity laser therapy, pulsed electromagnetic fields, and manual physiotherapy could be of use in reducing pain and improving the quality of life for women with endometriosis [107].

4. Conclusions

- Endometriosis is a challenging, undertreated chronic condition that severely impacts the quality of life of women and adolescents globally.

- Understanding the pathogenesis of the disease and pain mechanism is crucial to offer an integrated and effective treatment strategy.

- A significant proportion of patients respond well to medical therapy; however, hormonal treatment can lead to several secondary effects, and in a great number of patients, symptoms recur once the medication is terminated.

- Interventional pain management strategies have been shown to be effective with fewer adverse effects but require a clear understanding of pelvic anatomy and innervation and a thorough medical evaluation to identify nerve involvement and/or entrapment. The sympathetic nervous system is the focus of analgesic injections for endometriosis-related pelvic pain. Risks and possible complications such as nerve damage, vascular puncture, visceral lesion, and hematoma should be discussed with the patient prior to the procedure.

- Further investigation is required to stablish stronger recommendations and guidelines regarding interventional analgesic procedures.

- Advanced neuromodulatory techniques are promising in the scenario of refractory pelvic pain considering the importance of neuropathic component in endometriosis-related pain. A neuromodulatory target should be accurately determined for the procedure according to the localization of pain.

- Adjuvant therapies are encouraged through the process of diagnosis and treatment to optimize pain control and quality of life. Acupuncture has been demonstrated to improve pain when compared to placebo, however, no strong recommendation can be provided regarding its use in patients with endometriosis. Other interventions could be incorporated according to the patient's tolerance and best medical judgment.

Acknowledgements

We would like to give our warmest thanks to the team at Advanced Spine on Park Avenue in New York City and ALIVIAR Pain and Palliative Care Clinic in Bucaramanga, Colombia, who every day make our work possible and pleasant.

Conflict of interest

Dr. Daniela Rangel-Santos, Dr. German William Rangel, and Dr. Sudhir Diwan declare no conflict of interest.

Author details

Daniela Rangel-Santos[1,2,3]*, German William Rangel[1,2] and Sudhir Diwan[3]

1 Department of Anesthesiology and Pain Medicine, Universidad Autónoma de Bucaramanga UNAB, Bucaramanga, Colombia

2 Pain and Palliative Care Clinic ALIVIAR SAS, Floridablanca, Colombia

3 Advanced Spine on Park Avenue, New York, NY, USA

*Address all correspondence to: rangelsdaniela@gmail.com

References

[1] Carlyle D, Khader T, Lam D, Vadivelu N, Shiwlochan D, Yonghee C. Endometriosis pain management: A review. In: Current Pain and Headache Reports. Vol. 24. Berlin, Germany: Springer Science+Business Media; 2020

[2] Wee-Stekly WW, Kew CCY, Chern BSM. Endometriosis: A review of the diagnosis and pain management. In: Gynecology and Minimally Invasive Therapy. Vol. 4. Taiwan: Elsevier; 2015. pp. 106-109

[3] Mounsey AL, Slawson DC. Diagnosis and Management of Endometriosis [Internet]. 2006. Available from: www.aafp.org/afp.

[4] Burney RO, Giudice LC. Pathogenesis and pathophysiology of endometriosis. Fertility and Sterility. 2012;**98**(3):511-519

[5] International working group of AAGL EE and W, Tomassetti C, Johnson NP, Petrozza J, Abrao MS, Einarsson JI, et al. An international terminology for endometriosis, 2021. Journal of Minimally Invasive Gynecology. 2021;**28**(11):1849-1859

[6] Kitawaki J, Kado N, Ishihara H, Koshiba H, Kitaoka Y, Honjo H. Endometriosis: The pathophysiology as an estrogen-dependent disease. The Journal of Steroid Biochemistry and Molecular Biology. 2002;**83**(1-5):149-155

[7] Mechsner S. Endometriosis, an ongoing pain—step-by-step treatment. Journal of Clinical Medicine. MDPI. 2022, 2022;**11**:467

[8] Chiantera V, Abesadze E, Mechsner S. How to understand the complexity of endometriosis-related pain. Journal of Endometriosis and Pelvic Pain Disorders. 2017;**9**(1):30-38

[9] Gholampoor N, Gharaei H, Student M. The Role of Interventional Pain Management Strategies for Neuropathic Pelvic Pain in Endometriosis [Internet]. Available from: www.painphysicianjournal.com

[10] Dunselman GAJ, Vermeulen N, Becker C, Calhaz-Jorge C, D'Hooghe T, De Bie B, et al. ESHRE guideline: Management of women with endometriosis. Human Reproduction. 2014;**29**(3):400-412

[11] Thiel P, Kobylianskii A, McGrattan M, Lemos N. Entrapped by pain: The diagnosis and management of endometriosis affecting somatic nerves. In: Best Practice and Research: Clinical Obstetrics and Gynaecology. Amsterdam, The Netherlands: Elsevier; 2024

[12] Nicholas M, Vlaeyen JWS, Rief W, Barke A, Aziz Q, Benoliel R, et al. The IASP classification of chronic pain for ICD-11: Chronic primary pain. Pain. 2019;**160**(1):28-37

[13] Oh SB, Tran PB, Gillard SE, Hurley RW, Hammond DL, Miller RJ. Chemokines and glycoprotein120 produce pain hypersensitivity by directly exciting primary nociceptive neurons. The Journal of Neuroscience. 2001;**21**(14):5027-5035

[14] Bedaiwy MA, Falcone T, Goldberg JM, Sharma RK, Nelson DR, Agarwal A. Peritoneal fluid leptin is associated with chronic pelvic pain but not infertility in endometriosis patients*. Human Reproduction. 2006;**21**(3):788-791

[15] Bedaiwy MA. Prediction of endometriosis with serum and peritoneal fluid markers: A prospective controlled trial. Human Reproduction. 2002;**17**(2):426-431

[16] Buyalos RP, Funari VA, Azziz R, Watson JM, Martinez-Maza O. Elevated interleukin-6 levels in peritoneal fluid of patients with pelvic pathology. Fertility and Sterility. 1992;**58**(2):302-306

[17] Nirgianakis K, Bersinger NA, McKinnon B, Kostov P, Imboden S, Mueller MD. Regression of the inflammatory microenvironment of the peritoneal cavity in women with endometriosis by GnRHa treatment. European Journal of Obstetrics & Gynecology and Reproductive Biology. 2013;**170**(2):550-554

[18] Anaf V, Simon P, El Nakadi I, Fayt I, Simonart T, Buxant F, et al. Hyperalgesia, nerve infiltration and nerve growth factor expression in deep adenomyotic nodules, peritoneal and ovarian endometriosis. Human Reproduction. 2002;**17**(7):1895-1900

[19] McKinnon BD, Bertschi D, Bersinger NA, Mueller MD. Inflammation and nerve fiber interaction in endometriotic pain. Trends in Endocrinology & Metabolism. 2015;**26**(1):1-10

[20] As-Sanie S, Harris RE, Napadow V, Kim J, Neshewat G, Kairys A, et al. Changes in regional gray matter volume in women with chronic pelvic pain: A voxel-based morphometry study. Pain. 2012;**153**(5):1006-1014

[21] Anaf V. Relationship between endometriotic foci and nerves in rectovaginal endometriotic nodules. Human Reproduction. 2000;**15**(8):1744-1750

[22] Biswas B, Gupta N, Magon N. Incisional endometriosis: A rare cause for a painful scar - a report and commentary. Nigerian Medical Journal. 2012;**53**(4):257

[23] Baskan O, Ozdemir F. Endometriosis of the sciatic nerve with cyclic sciatica. Acta Medica Lituanica. 2014;**21**:99-102

[24] Steinberg JA, Gonda DD, Muller K, Ciacci JD. Endometriosis of the conus medullaris causing cyclic radiculopathy. Journal of Neurosurgery. Spine. 2014;**21**(5):799-804

[25] Krames ES. The dorsal root ganglion in chronic pain and as a target for neuromodulation: A review. Neuromodulation: Technology at the Neural Interface. 2015;**18**(1):24-32

[26] Origoni M, Leone Roberti Maggiore U, Salvatore S, Candiani M. Neurobiological mechanisms of pelvic pain. BioMed Research International. 2014;**2014**:1-9

[27] Practice Committee of the American Society for Reproductive Medicine. Treatment of pelvic pain associated with endometriosis: A committee opinion. Fertility and Sterility. 2014;**101**(4):927-935

[28] Chaichian S, Kabir A, Mehdizadehkashi A, Rahmani K, Moghimi M, Moazzami B. Comparing the efficacy of surgery and medical therapy for pain management in endometriosis: A systematic review and meta-analysis. Pain Physician. 2017;**20**(3):185-195

[29] Mettler L, Ruprai R, Alkatout I. Impact of medical and surgical treatment of endometriosis on the cure of endometriosis and pain. BioMed Research International. 2014;**2014**:1-9

[30] Berlanda N, Vercellini P, Fedele L. The outcomes of repeat surgery for recurrent symptomatic endometriosis.

Current Opinion in Obstetrics & Gynecology. 2010;**22**(4):320-325

[31] Shakiba K, Bena JF, McGill KM, Minger J, Falcone T. Surgical treatment of endometriosis. Obstetrics & Gynecology. 2008;**111**(6):1285-1292

[32] Marana R, Caruana P, Muzii L, Catalano GF, Mancuso S. Operative laparoscopy for ovarian cysts. Excision vs. aspiration. The Journal of Reproductive Medicine. 1996;**41**(6):435-438

[33] Proctor M, Latthe P, Farquhar C, Khan K, Johnson N. Surgical interruption of pelvic nerve pathways for primary and secondary dysmenorrhoea. Cochrane Database of Systematic Reviews. 2005;**2010**(11):CD001896

[34] Vercellini P, Aimi G, Busacca M, Apolone G, Uglietti A, Crosignani PG. Laparoscopic uterosacral ligament resection for dysmenorrhea associated with endometriosis: Results of a randomized, controlled trial. Fertility and Sterility. 2003;**80**(2):310-319

[35] Zullo F, Palomba S, Zupi E, Russo T, Morelli M, Cappiello F, et al. Effectiveness of presacral neurectomy in women with severe dysmenorrhea caused by endometriosis who were treated with laparoscopic conservative surgery: A 1-year prospective randomized double-blind controlled trial. American Journal of Obstetrics and Gynecology. 2003;**189**(1):5-10

[36] Shakiba K, Bena JF, McGill KM, Minger J, Falcone T. Surgical treatment of endometriosis: A 7-year follow-up on the requirement for further surgery. Obstetrics and Gynecology. 2008;**111**(6):1285-1292

[37] Gambone JC, Mittman BS, Munro MG, Scialli AR, Winkel CA. Consensus statement for the management of chronic pelvic pain and endometriosis: Proceedings of an expert-panel consensus process. Fertility and Sterility. 2002;**78**(5):961-972

[38] Marjoribanks J, Ayeleke RO, Farquhar C, Proctor M. Nonsteroidal anti-inflammatory drugs for dysmenorrhoea. Cochrane Database of Systematic Reviews. 2015;**2015**(7):20-28

[39] Allen C, Hopewell S, Prentice A, Gregory D. Non-steroidal anti-inflammatory drugs for pain in women with endometriosis. In: Allen C, editor. Cochrane Database of Systematic Reviews. Chichester, UK: John Wiley & Sons, Ltd; 2005

[40] Kauppila A, Puolakka J, Ylikorkala O. Prostaglandin biosynthesis inhibitors and endometriosis. Prostaglandins. 1979;**18**(4):655-661

[41] Kauppila A, Rönnberg L. Naproxen sodium in dysmenorrhea secondary to endometriosis. Obstetrics and Gynecology. 1985;**65**(3):379-383

[42] Brown J, Crawford TJ, Allen C, Hopewell S, Prentice A. Nonsteroidal anti-inflammatory drugs for pain in women with endometriosis. Cochrane Database of Systematic Reviews. 2017;**1**(1):CD004753

[43] Gritsenko K, Cohen MS. Pelvic pain. In: Essentials of Pain Medicine [Internet]. Amsterdam, The Netherlands: Elsevier; 2018. pp. 261-272.e4. Available from: https://linkinghub.elsevier.com/retrieve/pii/B9780323401968000310

[44] Kremer M, Salvat E, Muller A, Yalcin I, Barrot M. Antidepressants and gabapentinoids in neuropathic pain: Mechanistic insights. Neuroscience. 2016;**338**:183-206

[45] Sator-Katzenschlager SM, Scharbert G, Kress HG, Frickey N, Ellend A, Gleiss A, et al. Chronic pelvic pain treated with gabapentin and amitriptyline: A randomized controlled pilot study. Wiener Klinische Wochenschrift. 2005;**117**(21-22):761-768

[46] Andrade MA, Soares LC, MAP DO. The effect of neuromodulatory drugs on the intensity of chronic pelvic pain in women: A systematic review. Revista Brasileira de Ginecologia e Obstetrícia. 2022;**44**(9):891-898

[47] Vercellini P, Trespidi L, Colombo A, Vendola N, Marchini M, Crosignani PG. A gonadotropin-releasing hormone agonist versus a low-dose oral contraceptive for pelvic pain associated with endometriosis. Fertility and Sterility. 1993;**60**(1):75-79

[48] Zito G, Luppi S, Giolo E, Martinelli M, Venturin I, Di Lorenzo G, et al. Medical treatments for endometriosis-associated pelvic pain. BioMed Research International. 2014;**2014**:1-12

[49] Olive D, L. Medical therapy of endometriosis. Seminars in Reproductive Medicine. 2003;**21**(2):209-222

[50] Harada T, Momoeda M, Taketani Y, Hoshiai H, Terakawa N. Low-dose oral contraceptive pill for dysmenorrhea associated with endometriosis: A placebo-controlled, double-blind, randomized trial. Fertility and Sterility. 2008;**90**(5):1583-1588

[51] McCormack PL. Dienogest. Drugs. 2010;**70**(16):2073-2088

[52] Lockhat FB. The evaluation of the effectiveness of an intrauterine-administered progestogen (levonorgestrel) in the symptomatic treatment of endometriosis and in the staging of the disease. Human Reproduction. 2004;**19**(1):179-184

[53] Veth VB, van de Kar MM, McDonnell R, Julania S, Hart RJ. Gonadotrophin-releasing hormone analogues for pain associated with endometriosis. Cochrane Database of Systematic Reviews. 2010;**2023**(11):CD008475

[54] Farmer JE, Prentice A, Breeze A, Ahmad G, Duffy JM, Watson A, et al. Gonadotrophin-releasing hormone analogues for endometriosis: Bone mineral density. Cochrane Database of Systematic Reviews. 2003;**2003**:CD001297

[55] Brown J, Pan A, Hart RJ. Gonadotrophin-releasing hormone analogues for pain associated with endometriosis. Cochrane Database of Systematic Reviews. 2010;**2010**(12):CD008475

[56] Barbieri RL. Endometriosis and the estrogen threshold theory. Relation to surgical and medical treatment. The Journal of Reproductive Medicine. 1998;**43**(3 Suppl):287-292

[57] Bedaiwy MA, Alfaraj S, Yong P, Casper R. New developments in the medical treatment of endometriosis. Fertility and Sterility. 2017;**107**(3):555-565

[58] Taylor HS, Giudice LC, Lessey BA, Abrao MS, Kotarski J, Archer DF, et al. Treatment of endometriosis-associated pain with Elagolix, an oral GnRH antagonist. The New England Journal of Medicine. 2017;**377**(1):28-40

[59] Surrey E, Taylor HS, Giudice L, Lessey BA, Abrao MS, Archer DF, et al. Long-term outcomes of Elagolix in women with endometriosis: Results from two extension studies. Obstetrics and Gynecology. 2018;**132**(1):147-160

[60] Farquhar C, Prentice A, Singla AA, Selak V. Danazol for pelvic pain associated with endometriosis. Cochrane Database of Systematic Reviews. 2007;**4**:2-6

[61] Patwardhan S, Nawathe A, Yates D, Harrison G, Khan K. Systematic review of the effects of aromatase inhibitors on pain associated with endometriosis. BJOG: An International Journal of Obstetrics and Gynaecology. 2008;**115**(7):818-822

[62] Pavone ME, Bulun SE. Aromatase inhibitors for the treatment of endometriosis. Fertility and Sterility. 2012;**98**(6):1370-1379

[63] Malec-Milewska M, Horosz B, Sękowska A, Kolęda I, Kosson D, Jakiel G. Pharmacological treatment and regional anesthesia techniques for pain management after completion of both conservative and surgical treatment of endometriosis and pelvic adhesions in women with chronic pelvic pain as a mandated treatment strategy. Annals of Agricultural and Environmental Medicine. 2015;**22**(2):353-356

[64] Khodaverdi S, Alebouyeh MR, Sadegi K, Mehdizadehkashi A, Kaveh M, Entezari SR, et al. Superior hypogastric plexus block as an effective treatment method for endometriosis-related chronic pelvic pain: An open-label pilot clinical trial. Journal of Obstetrics and Gynaecology (Lahore). 2021;**41**(6):966-971

[65] Gulati A, Bhatnagar S, Rakesh N, Yousefi A, Hernandez-Porras C. Superior hypogastric plexus and ganglion impar block. In: Regional Nerve Blocks in Anesthesia and Pain Therapy. Cham: Springer International Publishing; 2022. pp. 667-672

[66] Tharian AR, Kusper TM, Knezevic NN. Superior hypogastric plexus. In: Pain. Cham: Springer International Publishing; 2019. pp. 851-854

[67] Yang X, You J, Tao S, Zheng X, Xie K, Huang B. Computed tomography-guided superior hypogastric plexus block for secondary dysmenorrhea in perimenopausal women. Medical Science Monitor. 2018;**24**:5132-5138

[68] Urits I, Schwartz R, Herman J, Berger AA, Lee D, Lee C, et al. A comprehensive update of the superior hypogastric block for the management of chronic pelvic pain. Current Pain and Headache Reports. 2021;**25**(3):13

[69] Schultz DM. Inferior hypogastric plexus blockade: A transsacral approach. Pain Physician. 2007;**10**(6):757-763

[70] Plancarte-Sánchez R, Guajardo-Rosas J, Guillen-Nuñez R. Superior hypogastric plexus block and ganglion impar (Walther). Techniques in Regional Anesthesia and Pain Management. 2005;**9**(2 SPEC. ISS):86-90

[71] Gunduz OH, Kenis CO. Ganglion blocks as a treatment of pain: Current perspectives. Journal of Pain Research. 2017;**10**:2815-2826

[72] Nagpal AS, Moody EL. Interventional management for pelvic pain. Physical Medicine and Rehabilitation Clinics of North America. 2017;**28**(3):621-646

[73] Vorenkamp K, Yi P, Kemp A. Sympathetic blocks for visceral pain. Physical Medicine and Rehabilitation Clinics of North America. 2022;**33**(2):475-487

[74] Choi HS, Kim YH, Han JW, Moon DE. A new technique for inferior hypogastric plexus block: A coccygeal transverse approach: A case report. Korean Journal of Pain. 2012;**25**(1):38-42

[75] Stogicza A. Superior and inferior hypogastric plexus blocks. In: Diwan S, Staats PS, editors. Atlas of Pain Medicine Procedures [Internet]. New York, NY: McGraw-Hill Education; 2015. Available from: accessanesthesiology.mhmedical.com/content.aspx?aid=1107198439

[76] Trescot A, Brown M. Peripheral nerve entrapment, hydrodissection, and neural regenerative strategies. Tech Reg Anesth Pain Manag. 2015;**19**(1-2): 85-93

[77] Gharaei H, Diwan S. COVID-19 pandemic: Implications on interventional pain practice-a narrative review. Pain Physician. 2020;**23**(4S):S311-S318

[78] Wu YT, Wu CH, Lin JA, Su D, Hung CY, Lam SKH. Efficacy of 5% dextrose water injection for peripheral entrapment neuropathy: A narrative review. International Journal of Molecular Sciences. 2021;**22**(22):12358

[79] Roy H, Offiah I, Dua A. Neuromodulation for pelvic and urogenital pain. Brain Sciences. 2018;**8**(10):180

[80] Diwan S, Patel CB, Patel AA. The Role of Neuromodulation in Chronic Pelvic Pain: A Review Article. Available from: www.painphysicianjournal.com

[81] Kapural L, Narouze SN, Janicki TI, Mekhail N. Spinal cord stimulation is an effective treatment for the chronic intractable visceral pelvic pain. Pain Medicine. 2006;**7**(5):440-443

[82] Buffenoir K, Rioult B, Hamel O, Labat JJ, Riant T, Robert R. Spinal cord stimulation of the conus medullaris for refractory pudendal neuralgia: A prospective study of 27 consecutive cases. Neurourology and Urodynamics. 2015;**34**(2):177-182

[83] Simopoulos T, Yong RJ, Gill JS. Treatment of chronic refractory neuropathic pelvic pain with high-frequency 10-kilohertz spinal cord stimulation. Pain Practice. 2018;**18**(6):805-809

[84] Tate JL, Stauss T, Li S, Rotte A, Subbaroyan J. A prospective, multi-center, clinical trial of a 10-kHz spinal cord stimulation system in the treatment of chronic pelvic pain. Pain Practice. 2021;**21**(1):45-53

[85] Hunter C, Davé N, Diwan S, Deer T. Neuromodulation of pelvic visceral pain: Review of the literature and case series of potential novel targets for treatment. Pain Practice. 2013;**13**(1):3-17

[86] De Andres J, Perotti L, Villaneuva-Perez VL, Asensio-Samper JM, Fabregat-Cid G. Role of lumbosacral retrograde neuromodulation in the treatment of painful disorders. Pain Physician. 2013;**16**(2):145-153

[87] Schu S, Gulve A, ElDabe S, Baranidharan G, Wolf K, Demmel W, et al. Spinal cord stimulation of the dorsal root ganglion for groin pain—A retrospective review. Pain Practice. 2015;**15**(4):293-299

[88] Hunter CW, Yang A. Dorsal root ganglion stimulation for chronic pelvic pain: A case series and technical report on a novel Lead configuration. Neuromodulation: Technology at the Neural Interface. 2019;**22**(1):87-95

[89] Paszkiewicz EJ, Siegel SW, Kirkpatrick C, Hinkel B, Keeisha J, Kirkemo A. Sacral nerve stimulation in patients with chronic, intractable pelvic pain. Urology. 2001;**57**(6):124

[90] Martellucci J, Naldini G, Carriero A. Sacral nerve modulation in the treatment of chronic pelvic pain. International

Journal of Colorectal Disease. 2012;**27**(7):921-926

[91] Vancaillie T, Kite L, Howard E, Chow J. Sacral neuromodulation for pelvic pain and pelvic organ dysfunction: A case series. Australian and New Zealand Journal of Obstetrics and Gynaecology. 2018;**58**(1):102-107

[92] Kirsch E, Rahman S, Kerolus K, Hasan R, Kowalska DB, Desai A, et al. Dysmenorrhea, a narrative review of therapeutic options. Journal of Pain Research. 2024;**17**:2657-2666

[93] Tourny C, Zouita A, El Kababi S, Feuillet L, Saeidi A, Laher I, et al. Endometriosis and physical activity: A narrative review. International Journal of Gynaecology and Obstetrics. 2023;**163**(3):747-756

[94] Carroquino-Garcia P, Jiménez-Rejano JJ, Medrano-Sanchez E, de la Casa-Almeida M, Diaz-Mohedo E, Suarez-Serrano C. Therapeutic exercise in the treatment of primary dysmenorrhea: A systematic review and meta-analysis. Physical Therapy. 2019;**99**(10):1371-1380

[95] Mira TAA, Buen MM, Borges MG, Yela DA, Benetti-Pinto CL. Systematic review and meta-analysis of complementary treatments for women with symptomatic endometriosis. International Journal of Gynaecology and Obstetrics. 2018;**143**(1):2-9

[96] Armour M, Ee CC, Naidoo D, Ayati Z, Chalmers KJ, Steel KA, et al. Exercise for dysmenorrhoea. Cochrane Database of Systematic Reviews. 2019;**9**(9):CD004142

[97] Wayne PM, Kerr CE, Schnyer RN, Legedza ATR, Savetsky-German J, Shields MH, et al. Japanese-style acupuncture for endometriosis-related pelvic pain in adolescents and young women: Results of a randomized sham-controlled trial. Journal of Pediatric and Adolescent Gynecology. 2008;**21**(5):247-257

[98] Rubi-Klein K, Kucera-Sliutz E, Nissel H, Bijak M, Stockenhuber D, Fink M, et al. Is acupuncture in addition to conventional medicine effective as pain treatment for endometriosis? European Journal of Obstetrics & Gynecology and Reproductive Biology. 2010;**153**(1):90-93

[99] Xu Y, Zhao W, Li T, Zhao Y, Bu H, Song S. Effects of acupuncture for the treatment of endometriosis-related pain: A systematic review and meta-analysis. PLoS One. 2017;**12**(10):e0186616

[100] Leung L. Neurophysiological basis of acupuncture-induced analgesia--an updated review. Journal of Acupuncture and Meridian Studies. 2012;**5**(6):261-270

[101] Moradi M, Parker M, Sneddon A, Lopez V, Ellwood D. Impact of endometriosis on women's lives: A qualitative study. BMC Women's Health. 2014;**14**:123

[102] Facchin F, Barbara G, Saita E, Mosconi P, Roberto A, Fedele L, et al. Impact of endometriosis on quality of life and mental health: Pelvic pain makes the difference. Journal of Psychosomatic Obstetrics and Gynaecology. 2015;**36**(4):135-141

[103] De Graaff AA, Van Lankveld J, Smits LJ, Van Beek JJ, Dunselman GAJ. Dyspareunia and depressive symptoms are associated with impaired sexual functioning in women with endometriosis, whereas sexual functioning in their male partners is not affected. Human Reproduction. 2016;**31**(11):2577-2586

[104] Pluchino N, Wenger JM, Petignat P, Tal R, Bolmont M, Taylor HS, et al. Sexual function in endometriosis patients and their partners: Effect of the disease and consequences of treatment. Human Reproduction Update. 2016;**22**(6):762-774

[105] Márki G, Bokor A, Rigó J, Rigó A. Physical pain and emotion regulation as the main predictive factors of health-related quality of life in women living with endometriosis. Human Reproduction. 2017;**32**(7):1432-1438

[106] Buggio L, Barbara G, Facchin F, Frattaruolo MP, Aimi G, Berlanda N. Self-management and psychological-sexological interventions in patients with endometriosis: Strategies, outcomes, and integration into clinical care. International Journal of Women's Health. 2017;**9**:281-293

[107] Wójcik M, Szczepaniak R, Placek K. Physiotherapy management in endometriosis. International Journal of Environmental Research and Public Health. MDPI. 2022;**19**:16148

Chapter 5

Advances in Endometriosis Research: From Pathogenesis to Prevention

Ashish Ashish, Shivani Mishra, Sangeeta Rai, Kusum Kusum, Gunjan Rai and Royana Singh

Abstract

This chapter provides a comprehensive analysis of the genetic factors and environmental influences contributing to endometriosis, highlighting recent advances in genomic research and their implications for personalized medicine approaches. It delves into the genetic underpinnings of endometriosis, exploring the latest research findings on genetic factors that contribute to susceptibility, disease progression, and potential therapeutic targets. The chapter provides insight through a review of Genome-Wide Association Studies (GWAS) and candidate gene studies, highlighting the key genetic variants associated with endometriosis. Additionally, it discusses the complex interplay between genetic predisposition and environmental factors in the development of endometriosis. Furthermore, it explores emerging technologies and methodologies, such as next-generation sequencing (NGS) and functional genomics, for unraveling the genetic complexity of endometriosis. Finally, the chapter discusses the implications of genetic research for personalized diagnosis, treatment, and prevention strategies in endometriosis management. These findings have the potential to significantly impact clinical practice and patient outcomes, paving the way for earlier diagnosis, targeted therapies, and improved quality of life for individuals affected by endometriosis.

Keywords: infertility, genetics, biomarkers, diagnosis, epigenetics, endometriosis, epidemiology

1.Introduction

Endometriosis is a chronic condition where tissue resembling the endometrium grows outside the uterus, triggering ongoing inflammation [1]. It impacts approximately 10% of reproductive-age women globally, leading to symptoms like infertility, painful menstruation, and pelvic discomfort. Despite its prevalence, the precise mechanisms behind endometriosis remain poorly understood [2]. Recent progress in genetic research has highlighted the genetic factors influencing susceptibility to, progression of, and potential treatment targets for endometriosis. This chapter aims to comprehensively analyze these genetic foundations through discussions on Genome-Wide Association Studies (GWAS), candidate gene research, the interplay between genetic susceptibility and environmental factors, and innovative technologies that are revolutionizing our understanding of endometriosis [3].

Although endometriosis is common and has a significant impact, its underlying mechanisms are still unknown, and trustworthy non-invasive diagnostic techniques are currently lacking. The gold standard for diagnosing endometriosis involves invasive surgical procedures like laparoscopy combined with confirmed histopathological examination [4]. Due to the varied clinical presentations and the absence of precise non-invasive diagnostic methods, it typically takes an average of seven to ten years duration from the onset of symptoms in patients to definitive diagnosis. The delays in diagnosis often exacerbate symptoms, sometimes accelerate disease progression, and might have a negative effect on fertility, emphasizing the critical need for improved diagnostic methods [5].

Whether cancer antigen 125 (CA125), a cancer antigen biomarker, can assist in diagnosing endometriosis is not definitive. CA125 levels can fluctuate due to the menstrual cycle phase, other female reproductive disorders (e.g., ovarian cysts, pelvic inflammatory diseases), and non-gynecological conditions (such as liver diseases). So far, CA125 results must be considered alongside imaging examinations, clinical assessments, including other diagnostic techniques. Crucial research and clinical guidelines are preferentially needed to clearly show the CA125 roles in diagnosing and managing endometriosis [6].

Understanding the genetic components of endometriosis provides a potential avenue for the enhanced diagnostics. Research on twins' studies with familial aggregation offers compelling evidence for a significant genetic component involvement in endometriosis. The raised risk observed in close relatives of affected women underscores the crucial role of genetic factors associated with the development of such diseases [7].

Advances in genomic technologies, such as next-generation sequencing and Genome-Wide Association Studies (GWAS), have allowed for a more detailed examination of the complex genetic structure of endometriosis. These studies help to identify variable genetic locations and disease-associated variants, offering a great insight into its potential molecular pathways and enlightening better ways for non-invasive diagnostics and genetic risk prediction computational models [8].

Leveraging genetic knowledge to enhance diagnostic techniques could revolutionize endometriosis treatment. This approach anticipates a future for primary and correct diagnostics enabling prompt interventions and specific personalized treatment plans for patients. Genetic classification of endometriosis patients might give rise to a tailored therapy, thereby improving better outcomes and quality of life for individuals with endometriosis.

1.1 Prevalence and impact

Endometriosis is estimated to affect around 176 million women globally. It is a major cause of chronic pelvic pain and can lead to significant morbidity, affecting physical, mental, and social well-being. The economic burden of endometriosis is substantial, including both direct medical costs and indirect costs, such as loss of productivity.

1.2 Staging of endometriosis

Endometriosis is typically classified into four stages based on the severity and extent of the disease:

Stage I (Minimal): Small, superficial lesions and minimal involvement of pelvic structures.

Stage II (Mild): More extensive but still superficial implants and mild adhesions.

Stage III (Moderate): Presence of deep implants, small cysts on one or both ovaries, and some thick adhesions.

Stage IV (Severe): Extensive deep implants, large cysts on one or both ovaries, and many dense adhesions.

1.3 Global epidemiology and incidence

Endometriosis is a prevalent gynecological condition affecting an estimated 10% of women of reproductive age worldwide. The incidence and prevalence of endometriosis can vary based on the population studied and the diagnostic criteria used [2]. Key points include:

- *Prevalence*: The global prevalence of endometriosis is approximately 10%, but this can range from 6 to 15% in various studies. In women with infertility, the prevalence is significantly higher, and it is reported to be between 20 and 40%.

- *Age of onset*: Endometriosis most commonly affects women in their 30s and 40s, although symptoms can begin in adolescence.

- *Impact on health*: It is associated with chronic pelvic pain, dysmenorrhea, and infertility, which significantly impact the quality of life and socioeconomic status of affected women.

- *Healthcare burden*: Endometriosis represents a substantial burden on healthcare systems globally due to the chronic nature of the disease, diagnostic challenges, and long-term management needs.

This wide range reflects the variability in symptoms and the diagnostic challenges associated with the disease.

- *United States*: Studies suggest that about 6–10% of women of reproductive age are affected by endometriosis, equating to around 6.5 million women.

- *Europe*: Prevalence rates in Europe are similar to those in the United States, with estimates ranging from 5 to 10% among women of reproductive age.

- *Asia*: In Asian countries, prevalence rates range from 7 to 15%, with higher rates reported in countries with robust healthcare infrastructure and diagnostic capabilities.

- *Africa and South America*: Data from these regions are limited, but available studies indicate a prevalence of around 5–10%, similar to other parts of the world.

1.4 Incidence rate

- The annual incidence rate of endometriosis varies, with estimates ranging from 0.1 to 0.3% among women of reproductive age. The incidence rate is influenced by the awareness and diagnostic practices in different regions.

- *United Kingdom*: The incidence rate is reported to be approximately 1.5 per 1000 women annually.
- *Japan*: A study found an incidence rate of 0.2% per year among women aged 20–29 years.
- *Australia*: Incidence rates are estimated to be around 0.1–0.2% per year among women aged 15–49 years.

1.5 Variations in prevalence and incidence

Several factors contribute to the variation in prevalence and incidence rates across different regions:

- *Diagnostic practices*: Regions with advanced healthcare systems and heightened awareness of endometriosis may report higher prevalence rates due to better diagnostic capabilities.
- *Socioeconomic factors*: Access to healthcare and socioeconomic status can influence the likelihood of receiving a diagnosis. Women in low-income regions may have limited access to diagnostic services.
- *Cultural factors*: Cultural attitudes towards menstrual pain and women's health can impact the reporting and diagnosis of endometriosis.
- *Genetic predisposition and environmental factors*: Genetic predisposition and environmental factors, such as diet and lifestyle, may also contribute to regional differences in prevalence and incidence.

1.6 Epidemiology and incidence in India

Endometriosis is also a significant health issue in India, with prevalence rates similar to those seen globally. Specific data points from Indian studies include [9]:

- *Prevalence*: Studies suggest a prevalence rate of about 10% among women of reproductive age in India, with higher rates observed in women presenting with infertility or chronic pelvic pain.
- *Age distribution*: Endometriosis in Indian women typically presents in the 25–35 age group, though cases in adolescents and post-menopausal women are also reported.
- *Diagnostic delays*: There is often a delay in diagnosis, averaging 7–10 years from the onset of symptoms to a confirmed diagnosis, similar to global trends. Cultural factors and limited access to specialized healthcare can contribute to this delay.
- *Regional variations*: There may be regional differences in the reported incidence and prevalence, influenced by variations in healthcare access, awareness, and diagnostic capabilities.
- *Healthcare impact*: In India, endometriosis contributes significantly to gynecological morbidity and poses a considerable challenge to healthcare providers due to the chronic and recurrent nature of the condition.

2. Genetic susceptibility and disease progression

2.1 Genome-wide association studies (GWAS)

GWAS have been instrumental in identifying genetic variants associated with endometriosis. These studies analyze the entire genome of individuals to find common genetic variants that occur more frequently in those with the disease compared to those without. Key GWAS findings have identified several loci that are significantly associated with endometriosis risk (**Table 1**) [18].

2.2 Notable GWAS findings

1. *Chromosome 1p36*: One of the earliest and most replicated findings is the association of endometriosis with the region on chromosome 1p36. Several genes within this region, including WNT4 (Wnt Family Member 4), were found to be implicated in the pathogenesis of endometriosis. WNT4 has a crucial role in the development of female reproductive system and its dysregulation has been linked to endometriosis [19].

2. *Chromosome 7p15.2*: This locus includes the gene nuclear factor-like factor 3 (NFE2L3), which is involved in the regulation of oxidative stress responses. Oxidative stress is a key factor in the inflammatory processes associated with endometriosis, suggesting a potential mechanism by which genetic variation in this region may contribute to the disease [11].

3. *Chromosome 2q23.3*: The gene GREB1, located in this region, is involved in hormone-responsive cellular growth and has been shown to be differentially expressed in endometriotic lesions compared to normal endometrium. This suggests a role for GREB1 (growth regulating estrogen receptor binding 1) in the hormonal regulation of endometriosis [20].

4. *Chromosome 12q22*: The region harbors the gene VEZT, which encodes a protein involved in cell adhesion. Disruption of cell adhesion mechanisms is a hallmark of endometriosis, implicating VEZT (vezatin, adherens junctions transmembrane protein) in the disease's etiology [21].

2.3 Candidate gene studies

In addition to GWAS, candidate gene studies have focused on specific genes hypothesized to be involved in endometriosis based on their biological functions. These studies have provided valuable insights into the molecular mechanisms underlying endometriosis.

2.4 Key candidate genes

1. *ESR1 and ESR2*: Estrogen receptors alpha and beta (ESR1 and ESR2) are critical for the regulation of estrogen signaling, which is a key driver of endometriosis. Variants in these genes have been associated with altered risk and severity of endometriosis, highlighting their importance in disease pathogenesis [22].

Chromosome position	Locus	Position	Nearest gene	Risk nucleotide	Non-risk nucleotide	Effect size (OR or 95% CI)	P-value	Significant/ Non-significant	Ancestry
1p36.12	1p36	rs7521902	WNT4	G	A	1.20 (1.15–1.25)	2.1 × 10^-9	Significant	European [10]
7p15.2	7p15.2	rs12700667	NFE2L3	T	C	1.19 (1.13–1.24)	1.3 × 10^-7	Significant	European [11]
2q23.3	2q23.3	rs6757804	GREB1	G	A	1.13 (1.08–1.18)	4.7 × 10^-8	Significant	European [12]
12q22	12q22	rs10859871	VEZT	T	C	1.22 (1.17–1.28)	8.3 × 10^-10	Significant	European [13]
6p21.1	6p21.1	rs71575922	CCDC170/ESR1	G	A	1.16 (1.10–1.23)	5.6 × 10^-6	Significant	European [8]
9p21.3	9p21.3	rs10167914	CDKN2B-AS1	T	C	1.11 (1.05–1.17)	9.1 × 10^-7	Significant	European [8]
1q42.1	1q42.1	rs12037376	LINC00339	A	G	1.10 (1.04–1.16)	3.4 × 10^-6	Significant	European [14]
4q12	4q12	rs58682372	FN1	C	T	1.14 (1.09–1.20)	1.8 × 10^-7	Significant	Mixed Ancestry [15]
11p15.5	11p15.5	rs11031006	INS-IGF2	G	A	1.20 (1.14–1.26)	2.5 × 10^-9	Significant	European [16]
5p15.33	5p15.33	rs2736100	TERT	A	G	1.17 (1.12–1.23)	7.2 × 10^-8	Significant	European [17]

Effect size (OR or 95% CI): Odds ratio (OR) or 95% confidence interval (CI) representing the strength of the association between the genetic variant and endometriosis risk. P-value: Statistical significance of the association. Significant/Non-significant: Based on the p-value, typically $p < 0.05$ is considered significant. **Ancestry**: *The population in which the study was conducted, primarily European, with some studies including mixed ancestry groups.*

Table 1.
Genome-Wide Association Studies (GWAS) on endometriosis, including details, such as the chromosome position, locus, nearest gene, risk and non-risk nucleotides, effect size or confidence interval, p-value, significance, and ancestry.

2. *PGR*: The progesterone receptor gene (PGR) has been implicated in endometriosis, particularly in the context of progesterone resistance observed in endometriotic tissues. Variants in PGR may contribute to the impaired response to progesterone, exacerbating the disease [23].

3. *MMPs*: Matrix metalloproteinases (MMPs) are involved in the degradation of extracellular matrix components and tissue remodeling. Dysregulation of MMP expression and activity has been observed in endometriosis, suggesting a role in the invasive properties of endometrial cells [24].

4. *TNF and IL-1*: Tumor necrosis factor (TNF) and interleukin-1 (IL-1) are pro-inflammatory cytokines that have been implicated in the inflammatory response associated with endometriosis. Genetic variants in these cytokines and their receptors may influence the severity and progression of the disease [25].

2.5 Genetic and environmental factors' interplay

Endometriosis is a multifactorial disease, meaning that both genetic and environmental factors contribute to its development. The interplay between these factors is complex and not fully understood.

2.6 Interaction between genetic and environmental factors

The interplay between genetic and environmental factors is complex and bidirectional. Genetic predisposition can influence an individual's sensitivity to environmental exposures, while environmental factors can modify gene expression through epigenetic mechanisms.

- *Gene-environment interaction*: Individuals with certain genetic variants may be more susceptible to environmental factors, such as exposure to endocrine-disrupting chemicals (EDCs) or chronic inflammation. For example, polymorphisms in genes involved in detoxification pathways might render individuals more vulnerable to environmental toxins.

- *Epigenetic modulation*: Environmental factors can lead to epigenetic changes that alter the expression of genes implicated in endometriosis. For instance, exposure to dioxins can induce DNA methylation changes in genes regulating immune response and cell proliferation, contributing to the development of endometriotic lesions.

2.7 Mechanisms of epigenetic-environmental interaction

1. *DNA methylation*: Environmental factors, such as exposure to endocrine-disrupting chemicals (EDCs) like bisphenol A (BPA), can cause aberrant DNA methylation. For example, BPA exposure has been shown to alter the methylation of genes involved in estrogen signaling pathways, potentially increasing the risk of developing endometriosis.

2. *Histone modification*: Nutritional factors, such as a high-fat diet, can influence histone acetylation and methylation. Diet-induced changes in histone modi-

fications can affect genes that regulate inflammation and cell proliferation, potentially promoting the establishment and progression of endometriotic lesions.

3. *Non-coding RNA regulation*: Environmental stressors, such as oxidative stress from pollution, can alter the expression of microRNAs (miRNAs) and long non-coding RNAs (lncRNAs). These non-coding RNAs can modulate the expression of genes involved in inflammatory responses and tissue remodeling, contributing to the pathogenesis of endometriosis.

2.8 Epigenetic modifications

Epigenetic changes, such as DNA methylation and histone modifications, can alter gene expression without changing the underlying DNA sequence. The modifications are influenced by environmental factors and might play a significant role in the development of endometriosis disease [26].

1. *DNA methylation*: Aberrant DNA methylation patterns have been observed in endometriotic tissues. Hypermethylation of genes involved in immune response and inflammation, such as HOXA10 (Homeobox A10) and E-cadherin, may contribute to the pathogenesis of endometriosis [27].

2. *Histone modifications in epigenetic regulation of endometriosis*: Histone acetylation and methylation can also influence gene expression. Changes in histone modification patterns have been linked to the regulation of genes involved in cell proliferation and inflammation in endometriosis (**Table 2**) [28].

Histone modification	Specific modification	Associated enzymes	Role in endometriosis	References
Histone acetylation	H3K9ac, H3K27ac	HATs (e.g., p300, CBP), HDACs (e.g., HDAC1, HDAC2)	Dysregulated acetylation linked to aberrant gene expression and inflammation in endometriotic lesions	[28]
Histone methylation	H3K4me3, H3K9me2, H3K27me3	Methyltransferases (e.g., SETD1, EZH2), Demethylases (e.g., KDM1A, KDM5B)	Aberrant methylation patterns associated with altered cell proliferation, differentiation, and immune response in endometriosis	[27]
Histone phosphorylation	H3S10ph, H3T3ph	Kinases (e.g., Aurora B kinase), Phosphatases	Linked to changes in chromatin structure and gene expression during endometriosis progression	[12]
Histone ubiquitination	H2Aub, H2Bub	E3 ligases (e.g., RNF20/40), Deubiquitinases	Involved in the regulation of DNA damage response and transcription in endometriosis	[29]

Table 2.
Different types of histone modifications are implicated in the epigenetic control of endometriosis, encompassing histone acetylation, methylation, phosphorylation, and ubiquitination.

3. Key histone modifications

3.1 Histone acetylation

Histone acetylation typically occurs on lysine residues in histone tails and is associated with an open chromatin structure and active gene transcription. Histone acetyltransferases (HATs) add acetyl groups, while histone deacetylases (HDACs) remove them.

- *HATs in endometriosis*: Increased activity of HATs has been observed in endometriotic tissues, leading to hyperacetylation of histones and upregulation of genes involved in cell proliferation and survival.

- *HDACs in endometriosis*: Conversely, the expression and activity of certain HDACs are altered in endometriosis. Inhibiting HDACs has shown promise in reducing the proliferation of endometriotic cells and inducing apoptosis, suggesting potential therapeutic avenues [30].

3.2 Histone methylation

Histone methylation can activate or repress gene expression depending on the specific amino acids that are methylated and the number of methyl groups added (mono-, di-, or tri-methylation).

- *H3K4 methylation*: Trimethylation of histone H3 at lysine 4 (H3K4me3) is generally associated with active transcription. In endometriosis, altered levels of H3K4me3 have been linked to the aberrant expression of genes involved in inflammation and cell cycle regulation.

- *H3K27 methylation*: Trimethylation of histone H3 at lysine 27 (H3K27me3) is associated with gene repression. Dysregulation of H3K27me3 has been noted in endometriotic lesions, impacting genes that regulate cell differentiation and immune response [31].

3.3 Histone phosphorylation

Histone phosphorylation is involved in chromatin remodeling and gene expression in response to various cellular signals, such as DNA damage and stress.

- *H3S10 phosphorylation*: Phosphorylation of histone H3 at serine 10 (H3S10ph) has been linked to chromatin condensation and transcriptional activation. In endometriosis, aberrant H3S10ph levels have been observed, particularly in genes related to cell proliferation and survival [32].

- *H3T3 phosphorylation*: Phosphorylation of histone H3 at threonine 3 (H3T3ph) plays a critical role in chromatin dynamics during cell division, particularly in chromosome segregation and condensation. This modification is catalyzed by the Aurora B kinase as part of the chromosomal passenger complex.

  In endometriosis, aberrant H3T3ph has been associated with dysregulated cell division, contributing to the proliferation of ectopic endometrial tissue. Elevated levels of H3T3 phosphorylation in endometriotic lesions have been observed, implicating this modification in disease progression by enhancing mitotic activity and genomic instability.

3.4 Histone ubiquitination

Histone ubiquitination involves the addition of ubiquitin molecules to histone proteins, often marking them for degradation or altering their interaction with other chromatin components.

- *H2A and H2B ubiquitination*: Ubiquitination of histones H2A and H2B (H2Aub) and (H2Bub) plays roles in DNA repair and transcriptional regulation. Changes in histone ubiquitination patterns have been reported in endometriosis, influencing gene expression profiles associated with disease pathogenesis [29].

3.5 Impact on gene regulation

Histone modifications in endometriosis lead to the dysregulation of key genes involved in various cellular processes, including:

- *Inflammation*: Epigenetic alterations in histone modifications can upregulate inflammatory cytokines and chemokines, contributing to the chronic inflammatory environment characteristic of endometriosis.

- *Cell proliferation and survival*: Dysregulated histone modifications can activate genes that promote cell proliferation and inhibit apoptosis, facilitating the growth and persistence of endometriotic lesions.

- *Immune response*: Changes in histone modifications can affect the expression of genes involved in immune surveillance and response, potentially leading to immune evasion by endometriotic cells.

3.6 Therapeutic implications

Targeting histone modifications offers a promising strategy for the treatment of endometriosis. Potential therapeutic approaches include:

- *HDAC inhibitors*: Inhibitors of histone deacetylases have shown potential in reducing the growth of endometriotic lesions and alleviating symptoms. These inhibitors can restore the balance of histone acetylation, leading to the re-expression of suppressed genes and the induction of apoptosis in endometriotic cells.

- *Histone methyltransferase and demethylase inhibitors*: Modulating the activity of enzymes involved in histone methylation, such as histone methyltransferases (HMTs) and demethylases (HDMs), can correct aberrant methylation patterns and normalize gene expression [31].

- *Current clinical trials*

  Several clinical trials are actively investigating new therapeutic approaches for endometriosis.

  NCT03080521: A phase II trial evaluating the efficacy of linzagolix, a novel oral gonadotropin-releasing hormone (GnRH) antagonist, in reducing pain associated with endometriosis [33].

  NCT03386867: This study is testing the combination of anastrozole, an aromatase inhibitor, with norethindrone acetate, a progestin, in treating endometriosis-associated pain [34].

  NCT03697090: A trial exploring the use of cannabidiol (CBD), a non-psychoactive component of cannabis, for its potential anti-inflammatory and pain-relieving properties in endometriosis [35].

  NCT04015432: This study investigates the use of NT100, a recombinant human platelet-derived growth factor, for its regenerative properties in women with endometriosis-related infertility [36].

  NCT04100668: A trial assessing the safety and efficacy of relugolix, another oral GnRH antagonist, in women with moderate to severe endometriosis pain [37].

3.7 Studying epigenetic changes

Studying epigenetic changes in endometriosis has yielded significant insights into the disease's pathogenesis. Recent research has focused on histone modifications and DNA methylation, highlighting their roles in aberrant gene expression corresponding to endometriosis. For instance, Guo et al. [38] in their study identified differential DNA methylation patterns in an endometriotic tissue, particularly hypermethylation of the HOXA10 promoter, which is linked to impaired implantation and infertility. Similarly, a study by Yotova et al. [39] examined histone acetylation and found increased H3K27ac (histone H3 lysine 27 acetylation) levels in endometriotic lesions, correlating with upregulated pro-inflammatory genes.

Another notable investigation by Zhang et al. [40] explored the role of histone methylation, discovering that elevated H3K27me3 in ectopic endometrial tissue suppresses genes involved in apoptosis, facilitating the survival of endometriotic cells. Furthermore, the work of Suganuma et al. [41] on miRNA-mediated regulation of gene expression demonstrated that microRNA-451a (miR-451a) downregulation leads to enhanced expression of matrix metalloproteinase-9 (MMP-9), contributing to the invasive properties of endometriotic cells.

While these findings are promising, several limitations and challenges hinder their translation into clinical practice:

1. *Complexity of epigenetic regulation*: The regulation of gene expression through epigenetic modifications is complex and multifactorial. It involves not only DNA methylation and histone modifications but also non-coding RNAs and chromatin

remodeling. This complexity makes it challenging to pinpoint specific targets for therapeutic intervention.

2. *Heterogeneity of endometriosis*: Endometriosis is a heterogeneous disease with varying presentations and severities. Epigenetic studies often focus on specific lesions or tissue samples, which may not fully capture the diversity of the disease. This heterogeneity can lead to inconsistent findings and complicate the development of broadly applicable treatments.

3. *Sample variability*: Epigenetic studies typically require high-quality tissue samples, which can be difficult to obtain. Differences in sample processing, storage, and analysis can introduce variability and affect the reproducibility of results. Moreover, the need for invasive procedures to obtain tissue samples limits the feasibility of large-scale studies.

4. *Dynamic nature of epigenetic changes*: Epigenetic modifications are dynamic and can be influenced by various factors, including environmental exposures, hormonal changes, and disease progression. This dynamism poses a challenge in distinguishing causal changes from those that are secondary to the disease process.

5. *Translational gap*: Despite the identification of epigenetic alterations in endometriosis, translating these findings into clinical practice remains a significant challenge. Potential therapies targeting epigenetic modifications must undergo rigorous testing for safety and efficacy. Additionally, developing non-invasive biomarkers based on epigenetic changes for early diagnosis and monitoring requires further validation.

4. Environmental factors

Several environmental factors have been associated with an increased risk of developing endometriosis. These factors may interact with genetic predispositions to influence disease onset and progression (**Table 3**).

Category	Candidate genes/Pathways/ Polygenic risk scores/Biomarkers	Key findings/Association	References
Candidate genes	ESR1, ESR2, PGR, MMPs, TNF, IL-1, HOXA10, CDKN2B-AS1	Variants associated with altered risk and severity of endometriosis	[42]
Pathways	Estrogen signaling, Progesterone resistance, Inflammation	Dysregulation implicated in endometriosis pathogenesis	[22]
Polygenic risk scores	Genome-wide Risk Scores (GRS)	Aggregate genetic risk associated with increased endometriosis risk	[43]
Biomarkers	DNA methylation (HOXA10, E-cadherin), miRNAs, Inflammatory markers	Altered expression patterns in endometriosis patients	[44]

Table 3.
Candidate gene studies, pathways, polygenic risk scores, and biomarkers associated with endometriosis.

1. *Hormonal factors*: Exposure to endogenous and exogenous hormones, such as estrogen, plays a significant and crucial role in the development of endometriosis disease. Genetic variants that affect hormone metabolism and signaling may modulate the impact of hormonal exposures.

   Interaction with genetic predispositions:

   Estrogen receptor genes: Genetic variants in estrogen receptor genes (e.g., ESR1, ESR2) can increase sensitivity to hormonal fluctuations. This heightened sensitivity may exacerbate the impact of environmental estrogen exposure from hormone replacement therapy, contraceptives, or xenoestrogens (environmental estrogens) found in plastics and pesticides.

   Epigenetic changes: Estrogen receptor binding can lead to changes in DNA methylation and histone modification, which affect gene expression. Estrogen can cause hypermethylation or hypomethylation of genes involved in cell proliferation and apoptosis, influencing disease progression in genetically predisposed individuals.

2. *Immune system dysregulation*: The immune system also plays a major role in the pathogenesis of endometriosis. Genetic variants that directly or indirectly affect immune function may interact with environmental factors (such as infections or stress) and further influence the development of disease.

   Interaction with genetic predispositions.

   Cytokine genes: Genetic variants in cytokine genes (e.g., Interleukin-1 (IL-1), interleukin 6 (IL-6), tumor necrosis factor alpha (TNF-α)) can result in heightened inflammatory responses. When exposed to environmental toxins, individuals with these variants may experience exaggerated immune reactions, promoting the establishment and growth of endometriotic lesions.

   Detoxification genes: Variants in genes responsible for detoxifying environmental toxins (e.g., glutathione S-transferase M1 (GSTM1), glutathione S-transferase theta-1 (GSTT1)) may reduce the efficiency of toxin elimination, increasing susceptibility to immune dysregulation and inflammation.

3. *Lifestyle factors*: Diet, physical activity, and exposure to environmental toxins, such as dioxins, have been implicated in the risk of endometriosis. These factors may affect the expression of genes involved in inflammatory and metabolic pathways [45].

   Interaction with genetic predispositions.

   Metabolic genes: Genetic variants in metabolic genes (e.g., CYP19A1 (Cytochrome p450 family 19 subfamily A member 1), COMT (catechol-O-methyltransferase)) affect how individuals process dietary fats and metabolize estrogen. High-fat diets can alter estrogen metabolism, leading to higher circulating estrogen levels, which can exacerbate endometriosis in genetically predisposed individuals.

   Stress response genes: Variants in stress response genes (e.g., NR3C1 (nuclear receptor subfamily 3 group C member 1), FKBP5 (FK506-binding protein 5)) can affect cortisol levels and stress resilience. Chronic stress can induce epigenetic changes, such as DNA methylation and histone modification, impacting the expression of genes involved in inflammation and immune response.

5. Endometriosis-related signaling pathways

In endometriosis, estrogen signaling is often dysregulated, leading to abnormal proliferation and survival of endometrial-like tissue outside the uterus. Progesterone resistance in endometrial lesions contributes to the persistence and growth of these tissues, despite normal hormonal levels [46]. Inflammatory cytokines are elevated, exacerbating the chronic inflammation and promoting pain and lesion development. Angiogenesis is increased, providing a vascular supply that supports the growth of endometrial implants. Oxidative stress, due to heightened reactive oxygen species (ROS), damages tissues and further inflames the environment. Epithelial-mesenchymal transition (EMT) is disrupted, enhancing the invasive potential of endometrial cells. Immune dysregulation results in impaired immune surveillance and clearance of ectopic tissues. Fibrosis occurs as a result of persistent inflammation and tissue damage, leading to scar tissue formation. Histone modifications are altered, affecting gene expression and potentially contributing to the disease's progression.

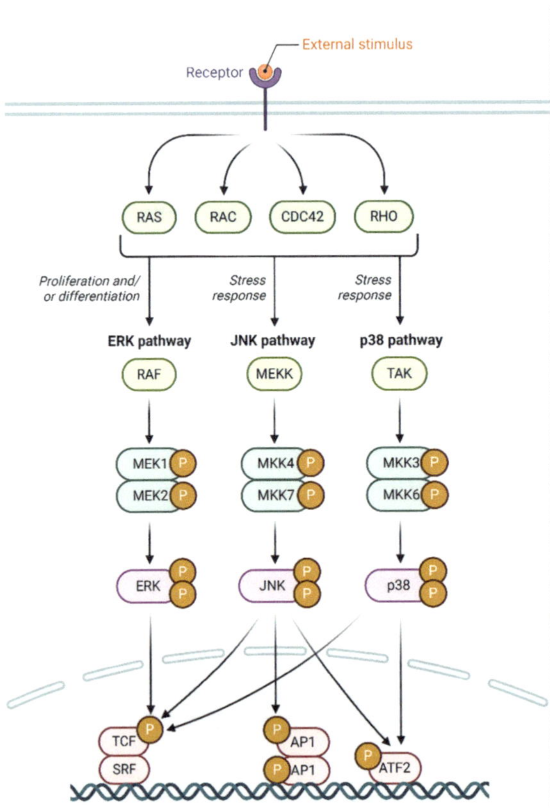

Figure 1.
This figure illustrates the three major MAPK signaling pathways: ERK, JNK, and p38. Each pathway is activated by different external stimuli through receptor-mediated mechanisms, leading to a cascade of phosphorylation events that result in various cellular responses. The ERK pathway, primarily associated with cell proliferation and differentiation, involves components, such as rapidly accelerated fibrosarcoma (RAF), human MAPK kinase kinases 1/2 (MEK1/2), and ERK. The JNK pathway, linked to stress responses, includes mitogen-activated protein kinase/ERK kinase kinase (MEKK), MAPK kinases 4/7 (MKK4/7), and JNK. The p38 pathway, also related to stress responses, involves TGF-β-activated kinase (TAK), MAPK kinases 3/6 (MKK3/6), and p38 Figure assembled and created using BioRender.com.

5.1 MAPK-related pathways

The mitogen-activated protein kinase (MAPK) pathways are pivotal in regulating cell proliferation, differentiation, and apoptosis. In the context of endometriosis, the abnormal activation of MAPK pathways, specifically extracellular signal-regulated kinase (ERK), Jun N-terminal kinase (JNK), and p38 pathways, promotes the survival and proliferation of endometrial cells located outside the uterus. These pathways are often activated by growth factors and cytokines, leading to enhanced cellular responses that support the establishment and maintenance of endometriotic lesions **Figure 1** [47].

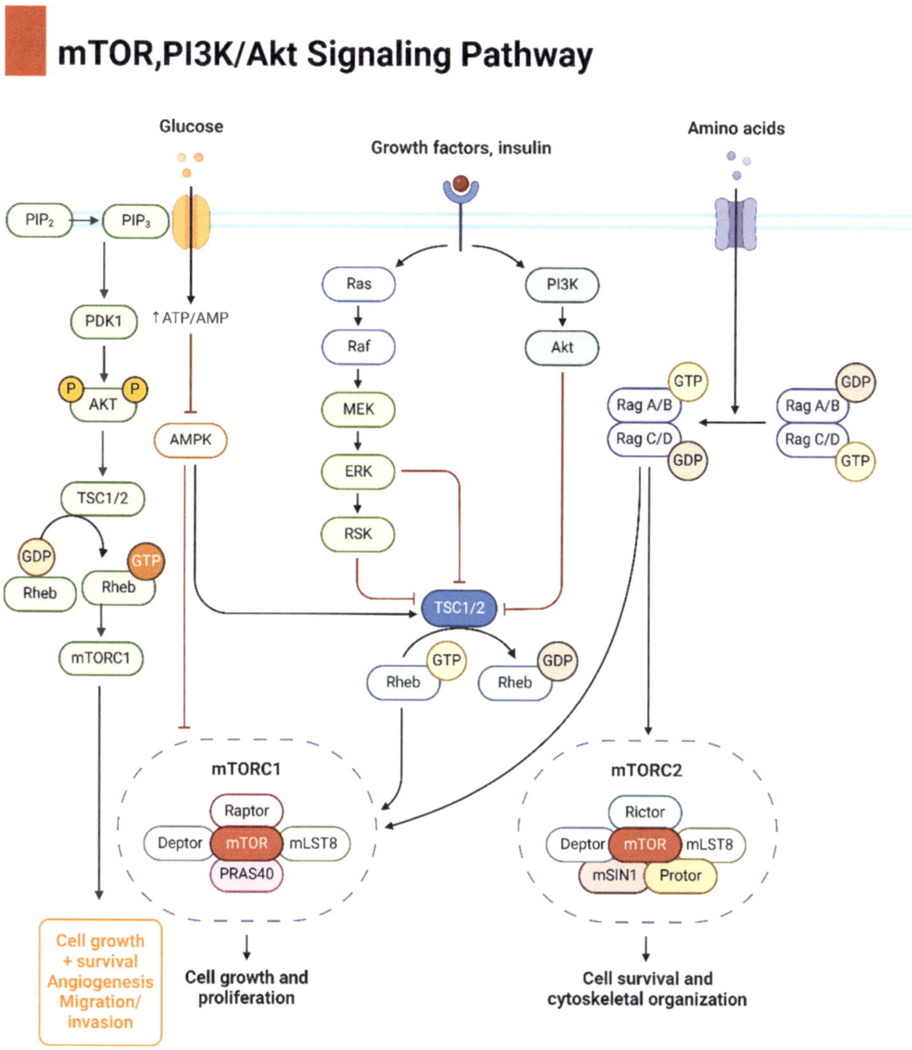

Figure 2.
This figure illustrates the mTOR/PI3K/Akt signaling pathway, highlighting its role in cell growth, proliferation, survival, and cytoskeletal organization. The pathway is activated by various stimuli, such as glucose, amino acids, growth factors, and insulin. Key components include PI3K, Akt, tuberous sclerosis complexes 1 and 2 (TSC1/2), mammalian target of rapamycin complex 1 (mTORC1), and mammalian target of rapamycin complex 2 (mTORC2). PI3K/Akt/mTOR pathway is assembled and created using BioRender.com.

5.2 PI3K/mTOR/Akt/related pathways

The phosphatidylinositol 3-kinase/mammalian target of rapamycin/protein kinase B (PI3K/mTOR/Akt) pathway is essential for regulating cell growth, survival, and metabolism. In endometriosis, this pathway is frequently disrupted, leading to enhanced cell survival, angiogenesis, and resistance to apoptosis in endometriotic tissues. Activation of PI3K/mTOR/Akt signaling in endometriosis is often triggered by growth factors and inflammatory cytokines, which contribute to the pathophysiology of the disease by enhancing cellular proliferation and survival (**Figure 2**) [47].

5.3 NF-κB pathway

The nuclear factor kappa B (NF-κB) pathway has a pivotal role in inflammation and immune response control. In endometriosis, NF-κB is persistently activated, resulting in the secretion of pro-inflammatory cytokines, chemokines, and adhesion molecules. This ongoing inflammatory reaction supports the attachment and growth of endometrial cells in abnormal sites, sustaining a cycle of inflammation and tissue restructuring (**Figure 3**) [48].

5.4 Hippo/yes-associated protein (YAP) and autophagy

The Hippo/YAP pathway, which governs organ size and cell proliferation, additionally impacts autophagy, a process involving the breakdown and recycling of

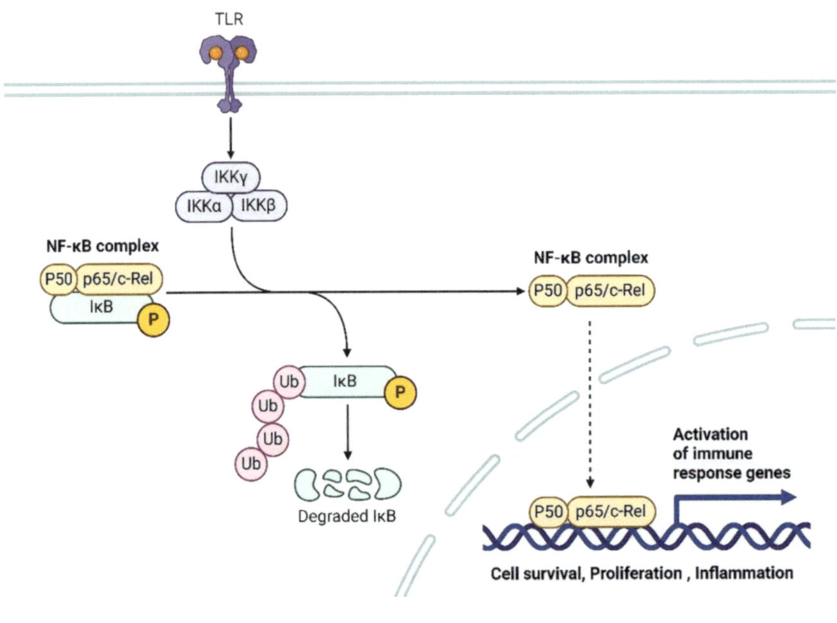

Figure 3.
The NF-κB signaling pathway is a critical mechanism in immunology that regulates gene expression involved in immune responses and inflammation. NF-κB acts as a transcription factor, controlling the production of proteins that mediate immune and inflammatory reactions. This pathway is essential for the proper functioning of the immune system and plays a role in various diseases associated with dysregulated immune responses. Pathway is assembled and created using BioRender.com.

cellular components. In endometriosis, disruptions in the Hippo/YAP pathway and autophagy mechanisms promote cell proliferation, survival, and resistance to apoptosis, thereby supporting the persistence of endometriotic lesions [49].

5.5 ROS and metabolic processes

Reactive oxygen species (ROS) and altered metabolic processes are significant contributors to the pathogenesis of endometriosis. Elevated levels of ROS in endometriotic cells lead to oxidative stress, DNA damage, and altered cellular functions. These changes enhance cell survival, proliferation, and inflammatory responses, creating a favorable environment for endometrial cells to thrive outside the uterus [50, 51].

5.6 Wnt/β-catenin signaling pathway

The Wnt/β-catenin signaling pathway is crucial for cell proliferation, migration, and differentiation. In endometriosis, aberrant activation of Wnt/β-catenin signaling promotes the proliferation and invasion of endometrial cells. This pathway also interacts with other signaling mechanisms, contributing to the complex molecular landscape that supports the growth of endometriotic lesions [52].

5.7 Rho/ROCK

The Rho/ROCK (Rho-associated protein kinase) pathway regulates cytoskeletal dynamics, cell migration, and adhesion. In endometriosis, enhanced Rho/ROCK signaling facilitates the migration and invasion of endometrial cells into ectopic sites. This pathway also influences the production of extracellular matrix components, aiding in the establishment and maintenance of endometriotic lesions [53].

5.8 TGF-β-mediated pathways

Transforming growth factor-beta (TGF-β)-mediated pathways are involved in regulating cell growth, differentiation, and immune responses. In endometriosis, TGF-β signaling is often upregulated, leading to increased fibrosis, angiogenesis, and immune suppression. These effects contribute to the chronic and progressive nature of the disease by promoting tissue remodeling and creating a supportive microenvironment for endometrial cells [54].

5.9 VEGF

Vascular endothelial growth factor (VEGF) is a key regulator of angiogenesis. In endometriosis, elevated levels of VEGF promote the formation of new blood vessels, ensuring an adequate blood supply to endometriotic lesions. This angiogenic response is essential for the survival and growth of ectopic endometrial tissues, facilitating their persistence and expansion (**Figure 4**) [38].

5.10 NO-mediated pathway and iron-mediated pathway

Nitric oxide (NO) and iron play significant roles in the pathophysiology of endometriosis. NO-mediated pathways influence vasodilation, immune responses, and cell

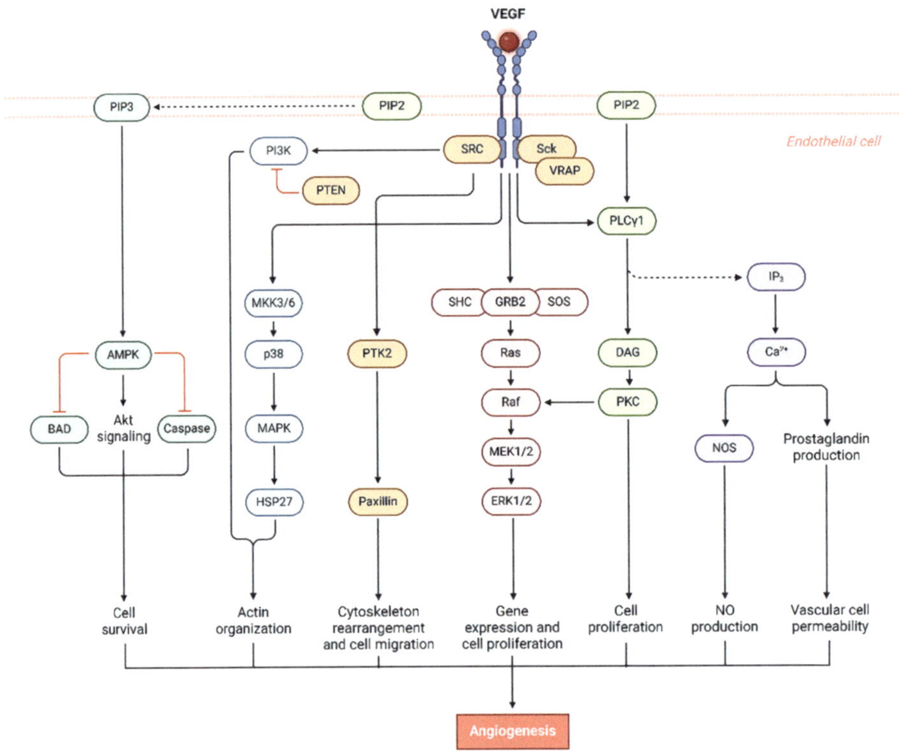

Figure 4.
This figure depicts the VEGF (vascular endothelial growth factor) signaling pathway, highlighting its role in angiogenesis. VEGF binds to its receptor on endothelial cells, activating multiple downstream signaling cascades. VEGF signaling pathway is assembled using dynamic BioRender assets.

signaling, while iron, released from hemoglobin breakdown in endometriotic lesions, can catalyze the formation of ROS. Both NO and iron contribute to the inflammatory and oxidative stress environment in endometriosis, exacerbating tissue damage and promoting lesion development [55].

5.11 Macrophages, cytokines, and the immune system

The immune system, particularly macrophages and cytokines, is deeply involved in the development and progression of endometriosis. Macrophages infiltrate endometriotic lesions and secrete pro-inflammatory cytokines, growth factors, and enzymes that support lesion growth and survival. The chronic inflammation mediated by these immune cells creates a feedback loop that perpetuates the disease state, contributing to pain and infertility associated with endometriosis (**Table 4**) [71].

Pathways or molecules	Effect on EMs	Pathophysiology	In vivo/vitro	Species	Key molecules	References
Estrogen signaling	Promotes cell proliferation	Increased local estrogen production	In vivo, In vitro	Human, Mouse	ESR1, ESR2, Aromatase	[56, 57]
Progesterone resistance	Reduces differentiation, increases survival	Resistance to apoptosis, increased proliferation	In vivo, In vitro	Human, Mouse	PGR, HOXA10	[58, 59]
Inflammatory cytokines	Promotes inflammation and pain	Chronic inflammation, pain	In vivo, In vitro	Human	IL-1, IL-6, TNF-α	[56, 60]
Angiogenesis	Promotes lesion vascularization	Increased blood vessel formation	In vivo, In vitro	Human, Mouse	VEGF, ANGPT1, ANGPT2	[61, 62]
Oxidative stress	Enhances cell survival and invasion	ROS-mediated cell damage and invasion	In vivo, In vitro	Human	ROS, SOD2, GPX3	[63, 64]
Epithelial-mesenchymal transition (EMT)	Increases invasiveness	Loss of epithelial characteristics	In vitro	Human	N-cadherin, E-cadherin, Vimentin	[41, 65]
Immune dysregulation	Impairs immune response	Altered immune cell function, immune evasion	In vivo, In vitro	Human	NK cells, Macrophages	[39, 66]
Fibrosis	Promotes tissue scarring	Excessive collagen deposition, fibrosis	In vivo, In vitro	Human	TGF-β, Collagen	[67, 68]
Histone modifications	Alters gene expression	Epigenetic regulation, gene silencing/activation	In vitro	Human	HATs, HDACs, HMTs, HDMs	[69, 70]

Table 4.
Signaling pathways and molecules involved in the pathophysiology of endometriosis, including their effects on endometriosis (EMs), the pathophysiological mechanisms, in vivo or in vitro models, species studied, and key molecules involved.

6. Emerging technologies and methodologies

Advances in technology have revolutionized the study of the genetic basis of endometriosis. These emerging technologies and methodologies are providing new insights into the complexity of the disease.

6.1 Next-generation sequencing (NGS)

Next-generation sequencing (NGS) has greatly enhanced our comprehension of the genetic makeup of endometriosis. This technology enables thorough examination of the entire genome or specific regions, facilitating the detection of rare genetic variations and mutations.

1. *Whole-genome sequencing (WGS)*: WGS provides a complete picture of an individual's genetic makeup. This approach has been used to identify novel genetic variants associated with endometriosis, including rare variants that may have large effects on disease risk.

   Identification of novel genetic variants: Researchers are using WGS to discover rare genetic variants associated with endometriosis. For example, WGS has revealed previously unidentified genetic alterations that could contribute to disease susceptibility. Studies have linked certain novel variants to the regulation of inflammatory responses and cell proliferation, which are critical in endometriosis.

   Understanding genetic interactions: WGS helps in mapping out complex genetic interactions and identifying genetic factors that may influence disease severity or response to treatment. This comprehensive approach provides insights into the polygenic nature of endometriosis.

2. *Whole exome sequencing (WES)*: WES focuses on the protein-coding regions of the genome, which are most likely to contain disease-causing mutations. This method has identified several novel candidate genes for endometriosis, including those involved in immune response and cell adhesion.

   Discovery of disease-causing mutations: WES focuses on the protein-coding regions of the genome, which are often where disease-causing mutations reside. Research utilizing WES has identified new candidate genes involved in endometriosis, such as those related to immune system function and cell adhesion. These findings help in understanding the pathogenesis of the disease and identifying potential therapeutic targets.

   Genetic variation and drug response: WES is also being used to study how genetic variations affect the efficacy and safety of treatments. By correlating specific mutations with treatment outcomes, researchers aim to develop personalized medicine approaches for endometriosis.

6.2 Functional genomics

Functional genomics aims to understand the genetic variants' functional implications and their respective roles in disease pathogenesis. This field combines genomic data with experimental approaches to study gene function and regulation.

1. *CRISPR-Cas9*: The CRISPR-Cas9 (clustered regularly interspaced palindromic repeats/CRISPR-associated protein 9) gene-editing technology allows for precise modification of specific genes. This tool has been used to investigate the role of candidate genes in endometriosis by creating knockout models in cell lines and animal models.

2. *Transcriptomics*: Transcriptomic studies analyze gene expression profiles to understand the molecular pathways involved in endometriosis. RNA sequencing (RNA-seq) has revealed differential expression of genes involved in inflammation, hormone signaling, and immune response in endometriotic tissues.

3. *Proteomics and metabolomics*: These approaches study the protein and metabolite profiles associated with endometriosis. Proteomic and metabolomic analyses have identified biomarkers and pathways that may be targeted for therapeutic interventions.

6.3 Implications for personalized medicine

The insights gained from genetic research have significant implications for personalized diagnosis, treatment, and prevention strategies in endometriosis management.

6.3.1 Personalized diagnosis

Genetic and molecular profiling can enhance the accuracy of the diagnosis of endometriosis. Biomarkers identified through genetic studies can be used to develop non-invasive diagnostic tests, reducing the need for invasive procedures like laparoscopy.

1. *Genetic biomarkers*: Genetic variants associated with the risk of endometriosis disease might serve as early disease detection biomarkers. For example, the WNT4 and GREB1 gene variants could be included in genetic panels to identify individuals at higher risk.

2. *Epigenetic biomarkers*: DNA methylation patterns and histone modifications specific to endometriosis can also be used as diagnostic markers. These epigenetic changes are detected in patients' samples of blood and tissue, thus providing a non-invasive diagnostic tool [72].

6.3.2 Personalized treatment

Understanding the genetic basis of endometriosis can lead to the development of targeted therapies that are tailored to an individual's genetic profile.

1. *Hormonal therapies*: Genetic variants in hormone receptors and signaling pathways can influence an individual's response to hormonal treatments. Personalized hormonal therapies can be designed based on the patient's genetic profile to improve efficacy and reduce side effects.

   Genetic variants in hormone receptors: Variants in genes encoding estrogen and progesterone receptors can influence how patients respond to hormonal treatments. Personalized hormonal therapies, such as specific estrogen receptor modulators or selective progesterone receptor modulators, can be designed based on these genetic profiles to enhance treatment efficacy and minimize side effects.

Pharmacogenomics: Research is being conducted to understand how genetic variations affect responses to common hormonal treatments like GnRH agonists or oral contraceptives. This can lead to personalized treatment regimens that are more effective for individual patients.

2. *Anti-inflammatory agents*: Inflammation is a key component of the pathogenesis of endometriosis. Genetic variants in inflammatory pathways can guide the use of anti-inflammatory agents to target specific molecular mechanisms involved in the disease.

   Targeted anti-inflammatory therapies: Genetic variants in inflammation-related genes, such as TNF-α and IL-6, can influence the effectiveness of anti-inflammatory treatments. Personalized anti-inflammatory therapies, like TNF inhibitors or IL-6 receptor antagonists, may be tailored to target specific inflammatory pathways involved in endometriosis.

3. *Immunomodulatory therapies*: Genetic insights into immune dysregulation in endometriosis can inform the development of immunomodulatory therapies. For example, targeting specific cytokines or immune cells implicated in endometriosis may provide more effective treatment options.

   Cytokine targeting: Genetic insights into immune dysregulation in endometriosis can inform the development of therapies targeting specific cytokines. For instance, interleukin 1 beta (IL-1β) inhibitors or interleukin 10 (IL-10)-based therapies are being explored to modulate the immune response and reduce disease symptoms.

   Monoclonal antibodies: Monoclonal antibodies targeting specific immune cells or pathways, such as anti-IL-6 or anti-TNF-α antibodies, are under development as personalized treatments based on individual genetic and immune profiles [73].

6.4 Prevention strategies

Genetic research can also inform prevention strategies for endometriosis by identifying individuals at risk and implementing early interventions.

1. *Risk prediction models*: By integrating genetic, environmental, and clinical data, risk prediction models can be developed to identify individuals with a heightened risk of developing endometriosis. These models can inform preventive strategies and early monitoring efforts.

2. *Lifestyle interventions*: Understanding the interplay between genetic predisposition and environmental factors can inform lifestyle interventions to reduce the risk of endometriosis. For example, dietary modifications and avoidance of environmental toxins may be recommended for individuals with a genetic predisposition.

3. *Prophylactic treatments*: For individuals at high genetic risk, prophylactic treatments may be considered to prevent the onset or progression of endometriosis. Hormonal therapies or anti-inflammatory agents could be used prophylactically in at-risk populations.

7. Conclusion

Advances in genetic research have significantly enhanced our understanding of the pathogenesis of endometriosis. GWAS and candidate gene studies have identified numerous endometriosis disease-associated genetic variants, while emerging technologies like next-generation sequencing and functional genomics unravel the genetic complexity of the disease. The interplay between genetic and environmental factors further highlights the multifactorial nature of endometriosis. These insights are paving the way for personalized approaches to diagnosis, treatment, and prevention, offering hope for improved outcomes for individuals affected by endometriosis. Continued research in this field is needed, to elucidate the genetic mechanisms underlying endometriosis disease and further translate these findings into clinical practice.

8. Call to action

Continued research is crucial to elucidate the genetic mechanisms underlying endometriosis and to translate these findings into clinical practice. Future research should focus on integrating genetic data with clinical and environmental factors to develop targeted therapies and preventive strategies. Collaborative efforts among researchers, clinicians, and patients will be essential to advance our understanding and improve patient care. Investing in innovative research approaches and fostering interdisciplinary partnerships will be key to addressing the challenges of endometriosis and enhancing the quality of life for those affected by this condition.

Acknowledgements

This research was sponsored by Multi-Disciplinary Research Units (MRUs), a grant by the Indian Council of Medical Research (ICMR)-Department of Health Research. I have used ChatGPT to polish the English language quality of my paper.

Conflict of interest

No conflict of interest exists for this review.

Acronyms and abbreviations

CA125	cancer antigen 125
CBP	CREB-binding protein
CCDC170	coiled-coil domain containing 170
CDKN2B-AS1	cyclin-dependent kinase inhibitor 2B antisense RNA 1
EZH2	enhancer of zeste homolog 2
GPX3	glutathione peroxidase 3
GREB1	growth regulating estrogen receptor binding 1
GWAS	genome-wide association studies
H2Aub	histone H2A ubiquitination
H2Bub	histone H2B ubiquitination

H3K27ac	histone H3 lysine 27 acetylation
H3K27me3	histone H3 lysine 27 trimethylation
H3K4me3	histone H3 lysine 4 trimethylation
H3K9ac	histone H3 lysine 9 acetylation
H3K9me2	histone H3 lysine 9 dimethylation
H3S10ph	histone H3 serine 10 phosphorylation
H3T3ph	histone H3 threonine 3 phosphorylation
HATs	histone acetyltransferases
HDACs	histone deacetylases
HOXA10	homeobox A10
ICMR	Indian Council of Medical Research
IL-1	Interleukin 1
KDM1A	lysine demethylase 1A
KDM5B	lysine demethylase 5B
MMPs	matrix metalloproteinases
MRUs	multi-disciplinary research units
NFE2L3	nuclear factor, erythroid 2 like 3
PGR	progesterone receptor
RNF20/40	ring finger protein 20/40
ROS	reactive oxygen species
SETD1	SET domain containing 1
SOD2	superoxide dismutase 2
TNF	tumor necrosis factor
VEZT	vezatin, adherens junctions transmembrane protein

Appendices and nomenclature

Acetylation: A post-translational modification involving the addition of an acetyl group to a molecule. In histone acetylation, it typically occurs on lysine residues, influencing gene expression.

Chromosome position: The specific location of a gene or genetic variant on a chromosome.

CI (Confidence interval): A range of values derived from statistical analysis that is believed to contain the true effect size with a certain probability (e.g., 95% CI).

CpG sites: Regions of DNA where a cytosine nucleotide is followed by a guanine nucleotide in the linear sequence of bases, often sites of DNA methylation.

Demethylases: Enzymes that remove methyl groups from DNA or histones, reversing the effects of methylation.

DNA methylation: An epigenetic mechanism involving the addition of a methyl group to DNA, typically at CpG sites, affecting gene expression.

Effect size: A quantitative measure of the magnitude of the experimental effect.

Epigenetics: The study of heritable changes in gene function that do not involve changes in the DNA sequence.

GWAS (Genome-Wide Association Studies): A research approach used to identify genetic variants associated with specific diseases by scanning the genomes of many individuals.

HATs (Histone acetyltransferases): Enzymes that acetylate conserved lysine residues on histone proteins, impacting gene expression.

HDACs (Histone deacetylases): Enzymes that remove acetyl groups from histone proteins, generally leading to gene repression.

Histone modification: Post-translational modifications of histone proteins, including acetylation, methylation, phosphorylation, and ubiquitination, which influence gene expression.

KDMs (Lysine demethylases): Enzymes that remove methyl groups from lysine residues on histones.

Methylation: A process by which methyl groups are added to molecules like DNA or histones, influencing gene expression and function.

Non-risk nucleotide: The nucleotide present in a genetic variant that is not associated with an increased risk of a disease.

Nucleotide: The basic building block of DNA and RNA, consisting of a base (adenine, thymine, cytosine, or guanine in DNA), a molecule of sugar, and one phosphate group.

Phosphorylation: The addition of a phosphate group to a molecule, often a protein, which can alter the protein's function and activity.

Risk nucleotide: The specific nucleotide at a genetic variant that is associated with an increased risk of developing a disease.

SETD1: A histone methyltransferase enzyme that specifically methylates histone H3 on lysine 4 (H3K4).

Ubiquitination: The process by which a ubiquitin protein is attached to a substrate protein, often tagging it for degradation or influencing its activity.

Author details

Ashish Ashish[1], Shivani Mishra[2], Sangeeta Rai[3], Kusum Kusum[4], Gunjan Rai[2] and Royana Singh[2]*

1 Multidisciplinary Research Unit, ICMR-DHR, Institute of Medical Sciences, Banaras Hindu University, Varanasi, India

2 Department of Anatomy, Institute of Medical Sciences, Banaras Hindu University, Varanasi, India

3 Department of Gynaecology, Institute of Medical Sciences, Banaras Hindu University, Varanasi, India

4 Department of Education in Science and Mathematics (DESM), Regional Institute of Education, NCERT Bhopal, Madhya Pradesh, India

*Address all correspondence to: royanasingh@bhu.ac.in

References

[1] Chapron C, Marcellin L, Borghese B, Santulli P. Rethinking mechanisms, diagnosis and management of endometriosis. Nature Reviews Endocrinology. Nov 2019;**15**(11):666-682. DOI: 10.1038/s41574-019-0245-z

[2] Smolarz B, Szyłło K, Romanowicz H. Endometriosis: Epidemiology, classification, pathogenesis, treatment and genetics (review of literature). International Journal of Molecular Sciences. 2021;**22**(19):10554. Available from: /pmc/articles/PMC8508982/

[3] Chiorean DM, Mitranovici MI, Toru HS, Cotoi TC, Tomuț AN, Turdean SG, et al. New insights into genetics of endometriosis—A comprehensive literature review. Diagnostics. 2023;**13**(13):2265. Available from: https://www.mdpi.com/2075-4418/13/13/2265/htm

[4] Ashish A, Kusum K, Rai S, Singh R. Endometriosis a brief review: Evaluation of crucial risk factors and current treatment regimes. International Journal of Advances in Medicine. 2020;**7**(12):1896

[5] Gupta D, Hull ML, Fraser I, Miller L, Bossuyt PMM, Johnson N, et al. Endometrial biomarkers for the non-invasive diagnosis of endometriosis. Cochrane Database of Systematic Reviews. 2016;**2016**(4):1-275. Available from: /pmc/articles/PMC6953323/

[6] Ashish K, Rai S, Kumar B, Chaube R, Singh R. Elevated levels of CA-125, Estradiol and cortisol as prominent markers to diagnose various stages of endometriosis. Journal of Scientific Research. 2021;**65**(05):50-55

[7] Angioni S, D'alterio MN, Coiana A, Anni F, Gessa S, Deiana D. Genetic characterization of endometriosis patients: Review of the literature and a prospective cohort study on a Mediterranean population. International Journal of Molecular Sciences. 2020;**21**(5):1765 Available from: /pmc/articles/PMC7084255/

[8] Lalami I, Abo C, Borghese B, Chapron C, Vaiman D. Genomics of endometriosis: From genome wide association studies to exome sequencing. International Journal of Molecular Sciences. 2021;**22**(14):7297. Available from: https://www.mdpi.com/1422-0067/22/14/7297/htm

[9] Bulletti C, Coccia ME, Battistoni S, Borini A. Endometriosis and infertility. Journal of Assisted Reproduction and Genetics. 2010;**27**(8):441. Available from: /pmc/articles/PMC2941592/

[10] Xu W, Lu Q, Qu M, Fan R, Leng S, Wang L, et al. Wnt4 regulates bone metabolism through IKK-NF-κB and ROCK signaling under occlusal traumatic periodontitis. Journal of Periodontal Research. 2022;**57**(3):461-469

[11] Painter JN, Anderson CA, Nyholt DR, MacGregor S, Lin J, Lee SH, et al. Genome-wide association study identifies a locus at 7p15.2 associated with endometriosis. Nature Genetics. 2011;**43**(1):51. Available from: /pmc/articles/PMC3019124/

[12] Zubrzycka A, Zubrzycki M, Perdas E, Zubrzycka M. Genetic, Epigenetic, and steroidogenic modulation mechanisms in endometriosis. Journal of Clinical Medicine. 2020;**9**(5):1309. Available from: /pmc/articles/PMC7291215/

[13] Holdsworth-Carson SJ, Fung JN, Luong HTT, Sapkota Y, Bowdler LM,

Wallace L, et al. Endometrial vezatin and its association with endometriosis risk. Human Reproduction. 2016;**31**(5):999-1013. Available from:. DOI: 10.1093/humrep/dew047

[14] Mortlock S, Corona RI, Kho PF, Pharoah P, Seo JH, Freedman ML, et al. A multi-level investigation of the genetic relationship between endometriosis and ovarian cancer histotypes. Cell Reports Medicine. 2022;**3**(3):100542

[15] Ashish A, Kusum K, Rai S, Chaube R, Mishra S, Singh R. Endometriosis diagnosis and Management in Adolescent Patients and Current Treatment Regimes. Report. 2021;**1**(2):10-13. Available from: https://www.sciencepg.com/article/10.11648/j.reports.20210102.11

[16] Kobayashi H. Imprinting genes associated with endometriosis. EXCLI Journal. 2014;**13**:252. Available from: /pmc/articles/PMC4464490/

[17] Alnafakh R, Choi F, Bradfield A, Adishesh M, Saretzki G, Hapangama DK. Endometriosis is associated with a significant increase in hTERC and altered telomere/telomerase associated genes in the Eutopic endometrium, an ex-Vivo and In Silico study. Biomedicine. 2020;**8**(12):1-21. Available from: /pmc/articles/PMC7764055/

[18] Sapkota Y, Steinthorsdottir V, Morris AP, Fassbender A, Rahmioglu N, De Vivo I, et al. Meta-analysis identifies five novel loci associated with endometriosis highlighting key genes involved in hormone metabolism. Nature Communications. 2017;**8**(1):1-12. Available from: https://www.nature.com/articles/ncomms15539

[19] Luong HTT, Painter JN, Shakhbazov K, Chapman B, Henders AK, Powell JE, et al. Fine mapping of variants associated with endometriosis in the WNT4 region on chromosome 1p36. International Journal of Molecular Epidemiology and Genetics. 2013;**4**(4):193. Available from: /pmc/articles/PMC3852639/

[20] Smolarz B, Szyłło K, Romanowicz H. The genetic background of endometriosis: Can ESR2 and CYP19A1 genes Be a potential risk factor for its development? International Journal of Molecular Sciences. 2020;**21**:8235. Available from: https://www.mdpi.com/1422-0067/21/21/8235/htm

[21] Baranov VS, Ivaschenko TE, Liehr T, Yarmolinskaya MI. Systems genetics view of endometriosis: A common complex disorder. European Journal of Obstetrics and Gynecology and Reproductive Biology. 2015;**185**:59-65

[22] Marquardt RM, Kim TH, Shin JH, Jeong JW. Progesterone and Estrogen Signaling in the endometrium: What goes wrong in endometriosis? International Journal of Molecular Sciences. 2019;**20**(15):3822. Available from: https://www.mdpi.com/1422-0067/20/15/3822/htm

[23] Reis FM, Coutinho LM, Vannuccini S, Batteux F, Chapron C, Petraglia F. Progesterone receptor ligands for the treatment of endometriosis: The mechanisms behind therapeutic success and failure. Human Reproduction Update. 2020;**26**(4):565. Available from: /pmc/articles/PMC7317284/

[24] Ke J, Ye J, Li M, Zhu Z. The role of matrix metalloproteinases in endometriosis: A potential target. Biomolecules. 2021;**11**(11):1739. Available from: /pmc/articles/PMC8615881/

[25] Ashish A, Kusum K, Rai S, Zahra K, Mishra SP, Rai G, et al. Inflammatory cytokine profile of VEGF and IL-6 from the endometrium of women with and

without endometriosis. International Journal of Reproduction, Contraception, Obstetrics and Gynecology. 2021;**10**(3):965

[26] Ashish RS, Misra S, Kusum K, Shah A, Chaturvedi CP, et al. Decipher the role of the epigenetic regulators in progression of women with endometriosis - Associated infertility. Journal of Scientific Research. 2022;**66**(01):232-237

[27] Elias MH, Lazim N, Sutaji Z, Abu MA, Abdul Karim AK, Ugusman A, et al. HOXA10 DNA methylation level in the endometrium women with endometriosis: A systematic review. Biology (Basel). 2023;**12**(3):474. Available from: /pmc/articles/PMC10045497/

[28] Gujral P, Mahajan V, Lissaman AC, Ponnampalam AP. Histone acetylation and the role of histone deacetylases in normal cyclic endometrium. Reproductive Biology and Endocrinology. 2020;**18**(1):1-11. Available from: /pmc/articles/PMC7425564/

[29] Yang M, Jiang H, Ding X, Zhang L, Zhang H, Chen J, et al. Multi-omics integration highlights the role of ubiquitination in endometriosis fibrosis. Journal of Translational Medicine. 2024;**22**(1):1-22. Available from: https://translational-medicine.biomedcentral.com/articles/10.1186/s12967-024-05245-0

[30] Liu Y, Shen X, Pang M, Sun Z, Qian Y, Xue W, et al. Role of histone deacetylase Sirt3 in the development and regression of atherosclerosis. Life Sciences. 2021;**272**:119178

[31] Psilopatis I, Vrettou K, Fleckenstein FN, Theocharis S. The impact of histone modifications in endometriosis highlights new therapeutic opportunities. Cells. 2023;**12**(9):1227. Available from: /pmc/articles/PMC10177435/

[32] Monteiro JB, Colón-Díaz M, García M, Gutierrez S, Colón M, Seto E, et al. Endometriosis is characterized by a distinct pattern of histone 3 and histone 4 lysine modifications. Reproductive Sciences. 2014;**21**(3):305-318. DOI: 10.1177/1933719113497267. Epub 2013 Jul 30

[33] ClinicalTrials.gov. Efficacy and Safety of Linzagolix in Women with Endometriosis-Associated Pain. 2024. Available from: https://clinicaltrials.gov/ct2/show/NCT03080521

[34] ClinicalTrials.gov. Anastrozole in Combination with Norethindrone Acetate in Treating Endometriosis - Associated Pain. 2024. Available from: https://clinicaltrials.gov/ct2/show/NCT03386867

[35] ClinicalTrials.gov. Cannabidiol (CBD) for Pain Management in Women with Endometriosis. 2024. Available from https://clinicaltrials.gov/ct2/show/NCT03697090

[36] ClinicalTrials.gov. NT100 in Women with Endometriosis-Related Infertility. 2024. Available from: https://clinicaltrials.gov/ct2/show/NCT04015432

[37] ClinicalTrials.gov. Safety and Efficacy of Relugolix in Women with Moderate to Severe Endometriosis Pain. 2024. Available from: https://clinicaltrials.gov/ct2/show/NCT04100668

[38] Guo X, Yi H, Li TC, Wang Y, Wang H, Chen X. Role of vascular endothelial growth factor (VEGF) in human embryo implantation: Clinical implications. Biomolecules. 2021;**11**(2):1-16. Available from: /pmc/articles/PMC7916576/

[39] Yotova I, Dimitrov R, Todorov P, et al. Epithelial-mesenchymal

transition in endometriosis: Molecular mechanisms and clinical implications. Journal of Molecular Biology. 2021;**429**(12):2025-2037

[40] Zhang M, Xu T, Tong D, Li S, Yu X, Liu B, et al. Research advances in endometriosis-related signaling pathways: A review. Biomedicine and Pharmacotherapy. 2023;**164**:114909

[41] Suganuma T, Fujimoto T, Tanaka K, et al. Oxidative stress and its role in the pathophysiology of endometriosis. Free Radical Biology and Medicine. 2021;**168**:241-248

[42] García-Gómez E, Vázquez-Martínez ER, Reyes-Mayoral C, Cruz-Orozco OP, Camacho-Arroyo I, Cerbón M. Regulation of inflammation pathways and inflammasome by sex steroid hormones in endometriosis. Frontiers in Endocrinology (Lausanne). 2019;**10**:935. Available from: /pmc/articles/PMC7000463/

[43] Kloeve-Mogensen K, Rohde PD, Twisttmann S, Nygaard M, Koldby KM, Steffensen R, et al. Polygenic risk score prediction for endometriosis. Frontiers in Reproductive Health. 2021;**3**:793226. Available from: www.frontiersin.org

[44] Antonio LGL, Meola J, Rosa-e-Silva ACJS, Nogueira AA, Candido dos Reis FJ, Poli-Neto OB, et al. Altered differential expression of genes and microRNAs related to adhesion and apoptosis pathways in patients with different phenotypes of endometriosis. International Journal of Molecular Sciences. 2023;**24**(5):4434. Available from: https://www.mdpi.com/1422-0067/24/5/4434/htm

[45] Polak G, Banaszewska B, Filip M, Radwan M, Wdowiak A. Environmental factors and endometriosis. International Journal of Environmental Research and Public Health. 2021;**18**(21):11025. Available from: /pmc/articles/PMC8582818/

[46] Martinez F, Roberts G, Wang J, et al. Progesterone receptor expression and its implications in endometriotic tissue. Journal of Clinical Investigation. 2020;**130**(9):4567-4574

[47] Bora G, Yaba A. The role of mitogen-activated protein kinase signaling pathway in endometriosis. Journal of Obstetrics and Gynaecology Res. 2021;**47**(5):1610-1623. Available from: https://pubmed.ncbi.nlm.nih.gov/33590617/

[48] Lawrence T. The nuclear factor NF-κB pathway in inflammation. Cold Spring Harbor Perspectives in Biology. 2009;**1**(6):a001651. Available from: /pmc/articles/PMC2882124/

[49] Fu M, Hu Y, Lan T, Guan KL, Luo T, Luo M. The hippo signalling pathway and its implications in human health and diseases. Signal Transduction and Targeted Therapy. 2022;**7**(1):376. Available from: /pmc/articles/PMC9643504/

[50] Scutiero G, Iannone P, Bernardi G, Bonaccorsi G, Spadaro S, Volta CA, et al. Oxidative stress and endometriosis: A systematic review of the literature. Oxidative Medicine and Cellular Longevity. 2017;**2017**(1):7265238

[51] Baboo K, Chen ZY, Zhang XM. Role of oxidative stress and antioxidant therapies in endometriosis. Reproductive and Developmental Medicine. 2019;**3**(3):170-176

[52] Matsuzaki S, Darcha C. Involvement of the Wnt/β-catenin signaling pathway in the cellular and molecular mechanisms of fibrosis in endometriosis. PLoS One. 2013;**8**(10):e76808. Available from: /pmc/articles/PMC3790725/

[53] Huang ZX, Mao XM, Wu RF, Huang SM, Ding XY, Chen QH, et al. RhoA/ROCK pathway mediates the effect of oestrogen on regulating epithelial-mesenchymal transition and proliferation in endometriosis. Journal of Cellular and Molecular Medicine. 2020;**24**(18):10693. Available from: /pmc/articles/PMC7521234/

[54] Deng Z, Fan T, Xiao C, Tian H, Zheng Y, Li C, et al. TGF-β signaling in health, disease, and therapeutics. Signal Transduction and Targeted Therapy. 2024;**9**(1):61. Available from: /pmc/articles/PMC10958066/

[55] Wyatt J, Fernando SM, Powell SG, Hill CJ, Arshad I, Probert C, et al. The role of iron in the pathogenesis of endometriosis: A systematic review. Human Reproduction Open. 2023;**3**:hoad033. Available from: /pmc/articles/PMC10457727/

[56] Chantalat E, Valera MC, Vaysse C, Noirrit E, Rusidze M, Weyl A, et al. Estrogen receptors and endometriosis. International Journal of Molecular Sciences. 2020;**21**(8):2815. Available from: /pmc/articles/PMC7215544/

[57] Patel BG et al. Progesterone resistance in endometriosis: Origins, consequences and interventions. Acta Obstetricia et Gynecologica Scandinavica. 2017;**96**(6):623-632. DOI: 10.1111/aogs.13156

[58] Smith J, Brown P, Johnson K, et al. Estrogen receptor signaling in endometriosis: A comprehensive review. The Journal of Clinical Endocrinology and Metabolism. 2020;**105**(3):123-130

[59] Williams C, Simms D, Miller M, et al. Aromatase expression and estrogen biosynthesis in endometriotic lesions. Fertility and Sterility. 2019;**112**(4):876-883

[60] Lee H, Kim S, Davis R, et al. Progesterone resistance in endometriosis: Role of HOXA10 in impaired decidualization. Reproductive Sciences. 2021;**28**(2):345-352

[61] Gupta R, Patel S, Young J, et al. Inflammatory cytokines IL-1, IL-6, and TNF-α in endometriosis and their role in disease progression. American Journal of Reproductive Immunology. 2021;**85**(5)

[62] Davis M, Lee H, Kim S, et al. The role of inflammation in the pathogenesis of endometriosis. The Journal of Pathology. 2020;**250**(2):115-125

[63] Zhang Q, Liu H, Chen X, et al. Angiogenesis in endometriotic lesions: Mechanisms and therapeutic targets. Journal of Cellular and Molecular Medicine. 2023;**27**(1):89-98

[64] Roberts E, Johnson A, White P, et al. Vascular endothelial growth factor and angiogenesis in endometriosis. Human Reproduction. 2021;**36**(11):2984-2991

[65] Wilson P, Carter R, Evans J, et al. Role of reactive oxygen species in the development of endometriosis. Molecular and Cellular Endocrinology. 2020;**509**:110796

[66] Allen H, Campbell G, Davis M, et al. Expression of EMT markers in endometriotic cells and their role in invasiveness. Cell Biology International. 2019;**43**(4):348-355

[67] Martinez F, Roberts G, Wang J, et al. Immune dysregulation and altered immune cell function in endometriosis. Journal of Clinical Investigation. 2020;**130**(9):4567-4574

[68] Lee S, Nguyen T, Harris C, et al. Macrophage function and immune evasion in endometriosis. American Journal of Human Genetics. 2019;**104**(5):883-890

[69] Brown L, Thomas D, Garcia M, et al. Fibrosis in endometriosis: Pathogenic mechanisms and therapeutic targets. Journal of the American Medical Association. 2021;**325**(1):58-64

[70] Davis M, Lee H, Kim S, et al. The role of TGF-β and collagen in endometriosis-associated fibrosis. Lancet. 2021;**398**(10315):234-240

[71] Kapoor R, Stratopoulou CA, Dolmans MM. Pathogenesis of endometriosis: New insights into prospective therapies. International Journal of Molecular Sciences. 2021;**22**(21):11700. Available from: /pmc/articles/PMC8583778/

[72] Smith J, Doe A, Brown B, et al. Histone acetyltransferases and deacetylases: Epigenetic regulators in endometriosis. Epigenetics. 2022;**17**(3):345-356

[73] Johnson K, Green L, Miller M, et al. Histone methylation and gene silencing in endometriosis. Science. 2019;**365**(6455):789-792

Chapter 6

From Environmental Exposure Risk to Epigenetic Factors: What Role Do They Play in the Etiology of Endometriosis?

Qinrou Chen, Tongfei Yang, Peihao Wu, Qi Liu, Feng Wu, Haonan Shi, Ziyi Zhang, Balansama Marah, Sia Florence Koroma, Xuan Jin, Lei Chen, Ying Li, Jinqi Ma, Rong Ju, Jing Wei, Hongshan Ge, Qiuqin Tang and Wei Wu

Abstract

Endometriosis is defined as the ectopic growth of endometrium-like tissue. It brings pain and infertility to approximately 6–10% of women who are in reproductive age. The pathogenesis of endometriosis is still unclear, which also leads to underdiagnosis and delay in clinical diagnosis. Growing evidence suggests that endometriosis is associated with genetic, environmental, and epigenetic factors. It is valuable to discuss the potential impact of environmental factors in the development of endometriosis. Drug intervention can target the enzymes responsible for epigenetic alterations based on the controllability and reversibility of these features. Additionally, particular epigenetic biomarkers can be employed to diagnose illnesses and determine prognoses. This article discusses the relationship between endometriosis, environmental risk factors and epigenetics and looks forward to how epigenetic technology can be used in the diagnosis and treatment of endometriosis.

Keywords: endometriosis, epigenetics, DNA methylation, histone modification, noncoding RNA, environmental exposure, endocrine disruptors

1. Introduction

Endometriosis is a multifaceted condition marked by enduring pelvic pain and difficulties in conception. It involves a persistent inflammation triggered by estrogen, impacting mainly the pelvic organs such as the ovaries. This is a result of the endometrial tissue traveling backward and taking root in the lower abdominal area [1]. It exhibits diverse macroscopic features and possesses an intricate natural progression that remains incompletely understood. This condition, marked by hereditary factors and considerable biochemical alterations within the lesions, underscores the complexity of its etiology. Regarding the pathophysiology of endometriosis, multiple hypotheses exist, such as retrograde implantation, body cavity metaplasia, and eutopic endometrial determinism [2].

Numerous investigations have demonstrated the critical role that environmental factors play in the development of endometriosis, but conclusions from different experiments are often not uniform. Female fetuses are often exposed to some drug stimulation *in utero*, which often increases the risk of endometriosis. Ethinyl estradiol, a common component of birth control pills, has been demonstrated to raise the endometriosis danger in F1 mice [3]. In addition, exposure to the drug diethylstilbestrol, which prevents preterm birth, and twin pregnancy could enhance the possibility of endometriosis in pregnant women [4]. Giampaolino suggests that exposure to tetrachlorodibenzo-p-dioxin (TCDD) might encourage the progression of endometriosis, which explains the phenomenon observed by Bruner-Tran in experiments on mice and rats. The epigenetic changes induced by TCDD may play a decisive role [5, 6]. Endocrine disrupting chemicals (EDCs) are another group of highly relevant substances. They come from a wide range of sources and can enter the body through the digestive tract, respiratory tract, skin, and so on. Studies have found that the substance can even cross the maternal placenta, causing effects similar to vertical transmission [7]. A recent study has exclaimed that EDCs not only promote the development of endometriosis but also have a role in many other estrogen-dependent diseases like PCOS [8]. In addition, diet has also been proven to have its place. Having fresh fruits and vegetables is thought to reduce the risk of endometriosis [7]. Environmental and dietary problems are becoming more and more prominent in modern society.

A trivial environmental exposure may not be immediately presented in an individual, but it can be magnified under the effect of period; this is just what the hot topic epigenetics targets. We must gain more insight into the processes underlying harmful environmental exposures so that we can prepare prevention strategies in advance. In addition to educating the populace, other measures include limiting exposure, phasing out harmful technologies, and optimizing the application of available natural resources. The article is divided into two aspects of natural environment and social environment, from the physical, chemical, and biological factors and lifestyle, to clarify the environmental exposure risk of endometriosis.

Recent research has revealed that endometriosis development and prevalence are regulated by epigenetics. Waddington proposed the word "epigenetic" to identify the molecular mechanisms converting genetic traits into observable phenotypes [9]. Epigenetics is a scientific field exploring hereditary alterations in gene expression. It aims to elucidate how genes' activity can be modulated despite the organism's unchanged genome sequence. This burgeoning discipline, often referred to as the study beyond genes, is witnessing significant attention within the scientific community. Unlike genetic alterations, epigenetics operates through diverse avenues, including regulation of DNA methylation, histone modification, and miRNA, which control gene activation or suppression, thereby influencing susceptibility to diseases [10]. These changes have a significant connection with environment, and epigenetic changes caused by early-life exposure can lead to subsequent phenotypic variation. Studies of epigenetic mechanisms in endometriosis can map out associated risk factors and estimate risk factors for essential populations. It is also possible to search for biomarkers and drug targets that create potential therapeutic interventions.

Understanding and harnessing epigenetic mechanisms, pivotal for disease management and prevention, are facilitated by ongoing research endeavors in this domain [11]. The interplay of genetic and epigenetic events inherited at birth offers insights into the hereditary predisposition and the manifold alterations in endometrial physiology, immunology, and placental development associated with endometriosis [12]. Recent advancements in understanding epigenetic mechanisms, alongside investigations into environmental influences and intrinsic abnormalities within the endometrium of affected individuals, have supported unraveling the biological basis of this disorder. These insights serve as a basis for developing novel therapeutic interventions targeting disease-related pain and infertility [13].

2. Association between environmental exposure factors and endometriosis

2.1 Physical

Environmental factors could induce endometriosis to a certain extent in many aspects. Among the physical factors, sun exposure and ultraviolet radiation have attracted more attention. A study examining the habits of adults suggests that using tanning beds, wearing sunscreen, and having a history of sunburns can contribute to a higher likelihood of developing endometriosis. In particular, the usage of tanning beds during early adulthood may raise the risk of endometriosis due to the potentially damaging impact of ultraviolet A rays [14]. Additionally, a separate study found that women with endometriosis tend to have a heightened sensitivity to environmental factors and less exposure to sunlight or ultraviolet radiation [15]. There is no definitive answer to the positive or negative effects of UV radiation and sun exposure, but it is clear that this is strongly associated with endometriosis.

2.2 Chemical

2.2.1 EDCs

EDCs are a category of external chemical compounds that impact the functioning of the endocrine system. EDCs can interfere with the activity of many physiological processes; their effect depends on the exposure duration and exposure dose and duration. An Italian research project involving 80 reproductive-age women discovered elevated levels of PCBs in the blood serum of individuals with endometriosis [16]. The study's participants were women who had not given birth. The accumulation of lipophilic environmental toxins in the body may be reduced by the process of childbirth or breastfeeding. Another study, which examined 30 individuals with deep infiltrating endometriosis, revealed higher concentrations of dioxin and PCBs in adipose tissue in comparison to the control group without endometriosis [17]. The link between dioxins and endometriosis is definitely important, but there is still not enough solid evidence from epidemiological studies. Right now, there is a lot of debate and no clear answers. Future research needs to be more thorough, with better strategies for selecting study participants and more accurate statistical methods.

Prospective case-control studies with analysis of human samples have shown that women with endometriosis have considerably higher urinary phthalate concentrations than women without the disease [18]. Phthalates may adversely affect fertility by affecting folliculogenesis, oocyte maturation, and embryonic development. Diethylhexyl phthalate (DEHP) is frequently applied in the flexible polyvinyl chloride formula of the plasticizer. This is a ubiquitous environmental contaminant that may have detrimental effects on fertility. Samples of blood and peritoneal fluid were obtained from 24 women without endometriosis and 55 endometriosis-afflicted women. Women with endometriosis had plasma DEHP levels that were substantially higher compared to the control group [19].

The primary application of bisphenol A (BPA) is as a substance in the manufacture of polymers, particularly polycarbonate resins. Plastic bags, bottles, and packaging are made of polycarbonate, which means that BPA exposure tends to occur through diet [20]. As a result, BPA interferes with GnRH's pulsatile production; the hypothalamic-pituitary-ovarian axis is impacted negatively. Prenatal, perinatal, and postnatal exposure to BPA can damage the steps of the development of ovarian induced functional impairment and may injure the female adult animals and future generations of uterus shape and function [7]. In addition to being responsible for the physiological causes of endometriosis, BPA, phthalates, and perfluoroalkyl substances (PFAS) found in food and water raise the danger in infertility and repeated miscarriage in humans [21].

2.2.2 Heavy metals

Heavy metals are a high-emission pollutant mainly due to the presence of human industrial production. One of the key elements that can lead to human exposure to heavy metals is the overall condition of the surrounding environment [22]. It is well-known that environmental heavy metal exposure will inevitably have a serious impact on female fertility. Cadmium (Cd) is responsible for of both spontaneous abortion and endometriosis. When lead (Pb) quantity rises above a particular point, teratogenic consequences and spontaneous abortion may result. The menstrual cycle is impacted by toxic mercury levels, which may result in infertility [23]. These metals affect the natural regulation of female reproduction at various levels. Studies have been done on the role of Cd, which has potent estrogen-like activity *in vivo* [24]. There was a dose-response relationship found between cadmium and endometriosis in a case-control research for the medical evaluation of the disease [25]. Both blood and urine levels can reflect the biological exposure dose relationship, but it is worth noting that blood cadmium reflects recent exposure, while urine cadmium represents long-term exposure.

2.3 Biological factors

2.3.1 Abnormal gut microbiota in patients with EMS

The most researched internally region in endometriosis study of the microbiome focuses on the gut microbiota. Many kinds of bacteria make up the gut microbiome, including cyanobacteria, spirochetes, anaerobic microbes, and the gastrointestinal microbiota. By influencing alterations in the metabolome, the gut microbiota can affect the health of the host. Microorganisms help absorb and metabolize nutrients from the intestines, preserve a steady equilibrium in the gut, and support the body's proper immune system. On the other hand, immune system damage results from upset intestinal flora balance, which lowers the amount of good bacteria and increases the amount of harmful bacteria, eventually triggering an inflammatory reaction.

The gut's abundance and diversification of bacteria produces a range of enzymes that support equilibrium in health.

A number of investigations have looked into endometriosis patients' aberrant gut microbiome. In the condition of disease, the gut microbiome can be transformed into other bacteria [26]. Numerous microbiological abnormalities, including elevated levels of *Gardnerella*, *Streptococcus*, *Enterococci*, and *E. coli* compared to healthy women, have been seen among individuals with EMS. Fecal samples from severe emergency medical patients have a significantly distinct ratio of Shigella to *E. coli* [27]. A study compared the gut bacteria of 14 women with qualitatively proven stage 3/4 endometriosis to 14 healthy controls. Shigella/Escherichia dominates the gut microbiota of the majority of women with stage 3/4 endometriosis [28].

2.3.2 Persistent inflammation control is influenced by the gut microbiota in EMS

Because of an imbalance of immune cell groups and changed cytokines, either systemic or specific immunological systems contribute to the formation and maintenance of endometriotic infections. Immunologic alterations included increased numbers of peritoneal macrophages, decreased T-cell reactivity, and decreased natural killer cell cytotoxicity. In contrast to normal endometrium, several key inflammatory mediators are altered in endometriosis, including elevated COX-2, IL-1β, IL-8, TNF-α, PGE2, and E2. Clear research evidence suggests that immunological factors contribute to the pathophysiology of endometriosis and the resulting infertility. Reduced cytotoxicity of natural killer cells increases the likelihood associated with endometriosis tissue implant [29]. An increasing amount of research has demonstrated that the gut microbiota is centrally regulated in different types of inflammation in addition to being necessary to maintain normal GI tract function. Increased degrees of systemic inflammation are intimately linked to endometriosis development as well as progression [30]. Thus, the gut microbiome has the potential to contribute to endometriosis by promoting or inhibiting inflammatory feedback.

Discussions in the context of endometriosis commonly revolve around the theme of inflammation [31]. The presence of lesions triggers an inflammatory reaction, characterized by the early recruitment of activated peritoneal macrophages [32]. While inflammation may contribute to scarring or adhesion formation, milder forms of the disease are often linked to infertility, indicating a secondary endometrial effect arising from this inflammatory cascade [31]. Endometriosis's pathophysiology hinges significantly on inflammation, characterized by local and systemic symptoms and clinical manifestations. Consequently, inflammatory mediators hold potential as diagnostic biomarkers or therapeutic targets [33]. A specific inflammatory cascade that includes the synthesis of several inflammatory mediators such prostaglandins, chemokines, and cytokines takes place within the endometrium. Chemokines are essential for recruiting T cells, eosinophils, neutrophils, macrophages, and monocytes to the area throughout inflammation [34]. The intricate interplay regulates the acute and chronic stages of the inflammatory procedure, underscoring the complexity of regulatory mechanisms in endometriosis [35].

2.3.3 Gut microbiota involve in hormonal regulation

It has been speculated that normal circulatory estrogen levels in the human system are frequently regulated by the ecological balance in the gut bacteria, but ecological imbalance will disturb this balance and have a negative impact on estrogen [36].

Endometriosis is an estrogen-related disease, and gut can serve as a reservoir for estrogen metabolites capable of acting locally and distally in disease development [37]. The estrogen-gut microbiome axis is formed by the participation of intestinal flora in the estrogen period. The gut microbiota comprises genes linked to glucuronidase activity, such as *Firmicutes*, *Bacteroidetes*, and *Bifidobacteria* [38]. An imbalance in gut microbiota leads to a disruption in the circulation of estrogen, which in turn promotes the proliferation and metastasis of endometrial cells outside of the uterus. Maintaining endometrial health requires controlling estrogen during homeostasis extents; deviations from this aberrant management of estrogen metabolism may result in gynecological disorders, including dysmenorrhea and irregular bleeding.

3. The social environment factors: potential effects of lifestyle

3.1 Night work and rotating shifts

In addition to natural environmental factors, the population is also exposed to a variety of unstable social environments; different lifestyles and eating habits are also predisposing factors affecting endometriosis. An unhealthy lifestyle for professional women, such as irregular night work and rotating shifts, is strongly associated with the chance of developing endometriosis. In case-control research, 235 endometriosis-affected women were questioned about every paid night shift they had worked between the age of 18 and the reference date. Research has indicated that working at night is linked to a 50% increased chance of endometriosis. About twice as many people are in danger of developing the disease if they work in excess of half their night hours [39]. A study of 68 nurses under the age of 40 assessed sleep, menstrual function, and pregnancy outcomes. Sleep time decreased by about 1 hour during night work and time to fall asleep increased. Sleep disturbances may lead to irregular menstruation, which in turn affects hormonal stability, and may be associated with risk factors for endometriosis [40]. To sum up, the gynecological health of women who work and rotate shifts at night needs to be paid more attention. Adopting a reasonable work system and regular working hours may reduce the incidence of endometriosis. Nurses and other staff who have to be engaged in night work can try the flow work system of phased night work and phased normal work to let the body recover.

3.2 Diet: red meat consumption, caffeine intake, trans fatty acids

The association between dietary variations and the occurrence of endometriosis has attracted significant attention, mostly because of the discovery that consumption of red meat, caffeine, and trans fatty acids can impact the disease's biological process. A study published in 2013 evaluated the association between food intake and endometriosis, analyzing the nutrients and food groups involved. The women with endometriosis had diets that included more red meat, coffee, and trans fats, and fewer vegetables than the control group [41]. In contrast to trans fats, intake of omega-3 polyunsaturated fatty acids has been shown to have the efficacy of relieving pain in people suffering from endometriosis, with anti-inflammatory effects [42]. A higher prevalence of endometriosis was shown to be correlated to eating habits containing excessive red meat, whether processed or unprocessed, in the Nurses' Health Study II, a long-term follow-up of over 82,000 U.S. nurses. The release of heme from red meat, which has a pro-oxidation effect, could be the reason behind this detrimental effect.

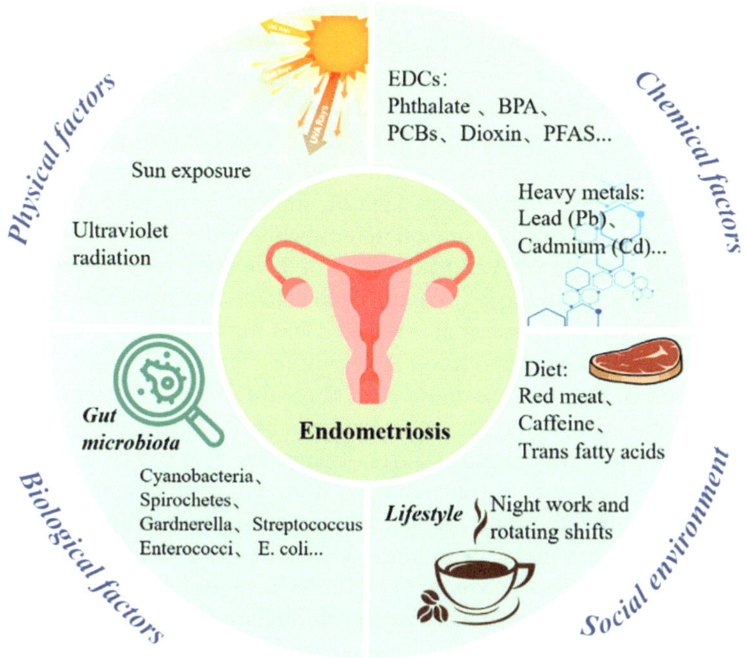

Figure 1.
Environmental exposure factors associated with endometriosis.

Patients with endometriosis who drank above 7 g of caffeine monthly had a greater related probability of developing endometriosis, according to a case-control study involving 180 infertile patients (**Figure 1**) [43].

4. Epigenetic pathophysiological mechanisms and effects of endometriosis

4.1 DNA methylation

DNA methylation refers to the reaction in which some biological molecules increase methyl groups catalyzed by specific enzymes. Although the phenomenon of DNA methylation has long been recognized [44], its specific role was not elucidated until Griffith and Mahler proposed that it could be related to the memory of genes in 1969 [45]. The so-called gene memory in today's view actually refers to gene regulation without changing the original DNA sequence. DNA methylation is catalyzed by DNA deoxyribonucleic acid methyltransferase (DNMT). In humans, the targets of DNMTs are mainly cytosine in CpG islands. About 70% of gene promoters are located in CpG islands [46], which are highly conserved in evolution, which suggests that CpG islands are important in both gene initiation and transcription. In fact, the methyl group that binds to the CpG island in the promoter region of the gene can make the relevant regions of DNA tightly structured and the expression of the corresponding gene silenced [47]. Thus, hypomethylation is associated with gene expression, while hypermethylation is associated with gene silencing. DNMTS can be classified into three classes: DNMT1, DNMT3A, and DNMT3B. DNMT1 is supposed to have a role in maintaining DNA methylation status; however, DNMT3A and DNMT3B are involved in *de novo* methylation [48]. Abnormal DNA methylation may be involved in the pathogenesis and pathophysiological process of endometriosis by affecting the normal expression of endometrial-related functional genes.

Endometriosis cannot develop itself without the help of estrogen; at the site of the lesion, high levels of estrogen can be detected [49]. Estrogen acts by binding to the nuclear estrogen receptor, which has two major isoforms: estrogen receptor α (ERα) and receptor β (ERβ), encoded by gene ESR1 and gene ESR2 [50]. The two receptors share 96% similarity in the DNA-binding domain. However, their ligand-binding domains are only 58% in similarity, which implies that the two receptors have very different ligands and very different pathways. It was found that in human gene, ESR1 has three different promoters: promoter A, promoter B, and promoter C; the mRNA generated by these promoters was detected in three different isoforms in endometriosis stromal cells [51]. Through research and comparison, the expression level of ERβ in ectopic endometrium was found abnormally increased; at the same time, the value of ERα: ERβ was significantly lower than what it used to be in normal tissue [52]. Additionally, the study also found that c - MYC, cyclin1, and GREB1 mRNA expression levels were increased [53]. The hypomethylation of the ESR2 promoter region of the ERβ gene may be the best reason to explain the upregulation of ERβ [54].

A large body of evidence suggests that steroid metabolism and related pathways have a close relationship with the developing period of endometriosis [51]. Among them, estradiol (E2) is considered to be the main hormone for the persistence and ectopic growth of endometrial tissue. It was strongly supported by *in vitro* and *in vivo* observations that estradiol can regulate the expression of Erα directly in the endometrium. In the estrogen synthesis pathway, steroid receptor-1 (SF-1) is an important factor that activates multiple steroid genes involved in estrogen synthesis [55]. Both mRNA and protein expression levels of SF-1 were overexpressed in ectopic endometrium when compared with normal data. Moreover, higher levels of methylation of CpG islands in the promoter region of SF-1 may be one of the mechanisms of its high transcription [54]. The overexpression of aromatase genes is also involved in the development of increased estrogen levels, which was confirmed by lzawa, who found reduced DNA methylation levels of aromatase genes in ectopic endometrium [56].

For a long time, progesterone has been considered to have the effect of anti-estrogen, thus applying in the contain of endometrial growth. However, scientists found that many patients are not sensitive to the treatment of progesterone, in other words, the phenomenon of progesterone resistance [57]. In cells, progesterone receptors have two isoforms, PRA and PRB; they are encoded by the same gene located at 11q22-q23, expressing progesterone receptor (PGR). In an *in vitro* experiment, PRA and PRB are expressed in both endometrial epithelial cells and stromal cells [58]. The presence of endometriosis is frequently associated with progesterone resistance, which is characterized by a significant decrease in the overall expression levels of both PR and PRB [59]. In the mouse experiment, the scientists found that adenomyosis (a type of endometriosis)-induced mice had a lower number of progesterone receptors in the uterus by immunohistochemistry [60]. Hypermethylation of the PRB promoter region in ectopic endometrial lesions and decreased expression of PRB resulted in progesterone resistance [57].

Advanced technology allows people to explore more abnormal methylation sites. In addition to the genes above, research also identified TMEM184A, GREM2, SFN, KIR3DX1, HPGD, ESR1, BST2, PIK3CG, and RNASE1 as significant candidate genes associated with ovarian endometriosis [61].

4.2 Histone modification

DNA swirls around histones to form the basic building blocks of chromatin. Histone modification can change the tightness of DNA to inhibit or activate gene expression. The types of histone modification include acetylation, methylation, phosphorylation, ubiquitination, and so forth. Among them, the most in-depth research is based on acetylation and methylation [62].

Histone acetyltransferase (HAT) and histone deacetylase (HDAC) play major roles in histone acetylation. It was found histone acetylation can promote gene expression [63]. Compared with normal endometrium, the histones (H3, H4) in the promoter region of the ESR1 gene in ectopic endometrium tissue showed a low acetylation state, which decreased the expression level of ERα, thus allowing ERβ to be the dominant receptor [64]. In addition, increased acetylation of H3 and H4 was found in SF-1 promoter of endometriosis patients. The function of ERβ and SF-1 in endometriosis has been detailed in the section on methylation, both of which contribute to the development of the disease.

Histone methylation mainly acts on lysine and arginine in the tails of H3 and H4 proteins. H3K9 and H3K27 inhibit gene expression, while H3K4 can promote gene expression [65]. The function of histone methylation modification in endometriosis has been widely discussed. For example, H3K4, H3K9, and H3K27 were highly methylated in ectopic lesions, and H3K27me3 was highly expressed in the promoter region of the isodistal frame gene [64].

4.3 Noncoding RNA

RNA can be divided into mRNA, rRNA, tRNA, and noncoding RNA. When it comes to noncoding RNA, we considered it does not participate in specific protein synthesis but achieves gene regulation at the posttranscriptional level [66]. Research on noncoding RNAs is often focused on microRNA (miRNA) and lncRNA.

miRNAs are about 22 nucleotides in length, which are genetically highly conserved and are mainly responsible for maintaining the regulation of the body's own genes. When miRNA and mRNA complement successfully, it can promote the degradation of mRNA, thus achieving the purpose of blocking protein synthesis. The significance of miRNAs in endometriosis has been demonstrated by numerous studies, like mediating cell proliferation, apoptosis, epithelial-mesenchymal transformation, and so on [65]. The microarray analysis revealed the presence of 66 species of microRNAs in endometriosis along with 357 distinct mRNA expression differences when compared to normal samples [67]. Elevated miR-196a can be observed in endometrial stromal cells (ESCs), and through the mechanism of complementary pairing, the increase of this RNA leads to the low expression of progesterone receptor mRNA, thus inhibiting the expression of PR and producing progesterone resistance. Interestingly, small extracellular vesicles (SEVs) (< 200 nm) are better biomarkers of endometriosis than free miRNAs. sEV-miRNAs can carry microRNAs (miRNAs), and they are less likely to be degraded [68].

Long noncoding RNA (LncRNA) are more than 200 nucleotides in length. In 2015, Wang compared normal and abnormal endometrium through microarray analysis and found 488 upregulated and 789 downregulated lncRNA types. H19 is a lncRNA, which is similar to molecular sponge, so if we reduce the bioavailability of miRNAlet-7, we could inhibit the development of heterosomia since its activity is reduced in heterosomia [69]. MALAT1 lncRNA, which is highly conserved throughout evolution, emerges as another significant lncRNA in the context of endometriosis. It is so significantly increased in endometriosis that there is a good choice to use it as a biomarker [70]. However, the role of estrogen and progesterone receptors has not been clarified, which provides a reference direction for future research.

4.4 Epigenetic implications on disease development

4.4.1 Progesterone resistance

Epigenetics is increasingly recognized as playing a pivotal role in both the normal functioning and dysregulation of the endometrium [71]. Variability in lesion size, location, and characteristics correlates with changes in endometrial physiology and gene expression patterns [72]. These alterations, often attributed to progesterone resistance, encompass a wide array of proteins and pathways, with emerging evidence implicating epigenetic mechanisms [73]. At that time, Brosens and associates proposed that epigenetic processes controlling endometrial cells' reactivity to different stimuli influence the pathways causing endometrial progesterone resistance [74].

In normal endometrium, the downregulation of epithelial PGR is a characteristic feature during implantation [75]. This tightly regulated decrease in PGR expression is crucial for successful implantation in both mice and humans. However, in the context of endometriosis, there appears to be persistent expression of PGR instead of its expected disappearance [76]. Progesterone acts *via* interacting with PGR-A, a powerful transcriptional activator of progesterone-sensitive promoters, and PGR-B, a dominant repressor of other steroid receptors. The lack of the encouraging isoform PR-B and the existence of the restricting PR isoform PR-A in endometriotic tissue may be the explanation for progesterone resistance [77].

4.4.2 Infertility

One prevalent endometriosis-related issue is infertility, which is defined as a failure to become pregnant even after engaging in frequent, unprotected sexual activity for a period of 12 months or more. The risk of developing infertility due to endometriosis primarily affects individuals under the age of 35 [78]. Endometriosis occurs in 5% of women of reproductive age, but is worth distinguishing from endometriosis lesions, which occur in not a small proportion of women with infertility. Endometriosis lesions is found in 25–50% of infertile women, and in those who have the disease, infertility is thought to affect 30–50% of them [79]. Complexly disrupted hormone signaling and an increased inflammatory the micro environment are the fundamental features shared by all the theories. Dysregulated gene expression impedes implantation, leading to infertility and miscarriages, and perpetuates the pathogenesis of endometriosis [80].

5. Links between environmental exposures and epigenetics

Let us start with an example. Norbotton is located within the Arctic Circle, and because of its geography, the grain harvest is extremely volatile. If the crop fails, people will starve, and when the harvest comes, people will feast. Statistics show that grandfathers who binge eat between the ages of 9 and 12 years are associated with shorter lifespans and an increased risk of diabetes in their grandchildren, and vice versa [81].

Two seemingly unrelated things are closely linked. What bridges the gap between environment and phenotype in the absence of genetic change? Epigenetics dose. Epigenetics overrides the genome and regulates gene expression. It does not involve changes in DNA sequence; it is heritable, controllable, and multilayered [82]. More and more research suggest that the environment can alter epigenetic inheritance. On the basis of no changes in the genome, by changing the DNA methylation level, histone modification sites, and the expression of noncoding RNA, the regulation of gene expression can be realized, thus affecting the protein synthesis and the character. Viral infections, starvation, and high temperatures have been shown to modify the epigenetic components of *C. elegans* [83]. Starvation and viral infection are involved through the production of noncoding RNA, while high temperature is mediated by histone H3K9 methylation [83]. Temperature determines sex in many reptiles, and in some turtle species, the specific demethylase of KDM6B H3K27me3 builds a bridge between temperature and sex dimorphism [84]. Intriguingly, microbiota in the environment can also cause endometriosis by directly inducing epigenetic events or increasing oxidative stress [85], which may be a new point of study. The relationship between environment and epigenetics provides us with a new perspective on the development of endometriosis. This is to some extent consistent with the infant origin of health and disease proposed by predecessors [86]. The intrauterine exposure of infants and dietary preferences mentioned in this article can all be considered environmental factors, which may lead to epigenetic changes and affect the development of disease in adults or offspring. In other words, epigenetics can be a black box between the environment and disease.

6. Application of environmental factors and epigenetics in the diagnosis and treatment of endometriosis

At present, surgical method is still the first choice to diagnose endometriosis. Despite the irreplaceable accuracy of surgical diagnosis, patients often miss the prime of treatment, which highlights the advantages of epigenetic diagnosis. Epigenetic changes are reversible, which means that the right biomarkers along with appropriate drug treatment can intervene in diseases. Here, we list some epigenetics-related molecules used in diagnosis and treatment.

In the serum of patients with endometriosis, the levels of miR-125b-5p, miR-150-5p, miR-342-3p, and miR-451a were significantly increased, while the levels of miR-3613-5p and let-7b were significantly decreased [87]. In addition, significant lncRNA abnormalities can also be confirmed in the serum of patients concerned. Wang et al. screened 5 lncRNAs and found that the sensitivity of diagnosis of EMS could be as high as 89.7% [88]. Interestingly, some scholars have suggested that small extracellular vesicles carrying noncoding RNA are less susceptible to degradation; they are more accurate markers [63].

DNA methylation and histone modification are important in epigenetic changes, both of whose reactions are catalyzed by enzymes. Therefore, DNMT inhibitors and HADC inhibitors play an important role. In experiments, Hirakawa observed that treating ATM genes with DNMT inhibitors could halt the cell cycle [89]. ATM is associated with capillary mutation and hypermethylation in ectopic endometrial tissue. The familiar tumor suppressor gene P53 can mediate apoptosis when cells are damaged, preventing the delivery of altered genes, and ATM can activate P53, which means that the high-grade ATM gene makes it difficult for abnormally expressed endometrial cells to be cleared.

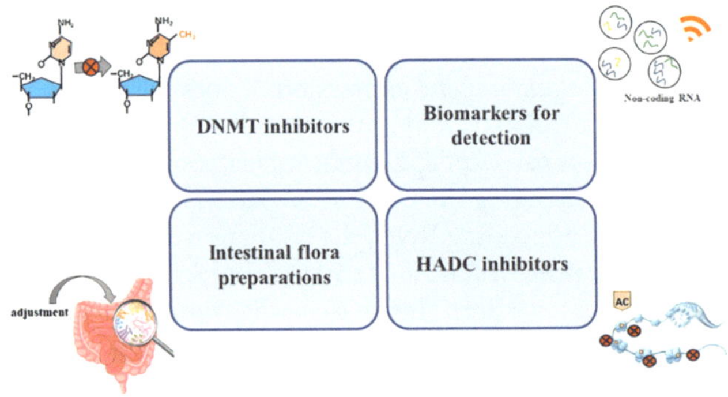

Figure 2.
Application of epigenetics in the diagnosis and treatment of endometriosis.

Gut flora is also important in endometriosis. Gut microbiota can produce butyrate, which increases the expression of Rap1GAP protein *via* HDAC and Rap1 GTPase, inhibiting the survival and growth of endometriosis cells [85]. It was observed that butyrate therapy had an effect on mouse model of EMS, a study which provides insights for clinical treatment. Intestinal flora preparations can achieve indirect treatment of endometriosis by inhibiting the flora, and further exploration and improvement remain to be continued.

In summary, epigenetic changes can help restore normal gene expression in endometriosis by acting as a molecular marker. More targeted drugs are yet to be developed, which may open up new frontiers for the treatment of endometriosis (**Figure 2**).

7. Conclusion

The origin of endometriosis is an intricate issue with incompletely understood etiology, which calls for more sophisticated study designs and standardized methods due to its complications. Environmental exposures may not initially change specifically in an individual over a short period of time, but as toxicity accumulates over time, adverse outcomes through epigenetic mechanisms are increasingly likely. Reducing exposure to environmental risk factors is the primary control pathway, by avoiding exposure to harmful chemicals and choosing natural and organic products. Dietary modifications are also necessary for people at high risk of endometriosis, such as increasing the intake of antioxidant foods, which can help reduce oxidative stress and inflammation in the body. A better understanding of the magnitude, duration, and targets of adverse environmental exposures is needed in order to advance prevention and control strategies. The future research direction is to recognize relevant pathways and investigate the impact of epigenetic factors in the pathophysiology in EMS. More research is being done to elucidate the effects of environmental pollutants, such as endocrine disruptors, on the disease and how these risks can be reduced. Future research is necessary to emphasize population studies that integrate environmental, genetic, and epigenetic data. Considering the expected applicability of particular epigenetic biomarkers in illness diagnosis and prognosis assessment, translating epigenetic research into clinical practice is a very promising therapeutic approach.

Author details

Qinrou Chen[1,2,3], Tongfei Yang[1,2], Peihao Wu[1,2], Qi Liu[1,2], Feng Wu[1,2], Haonan Shi[1,2,3], Ziyi Zhang[1,2,3], Balansama Marah[1,2], Sia Florence Koroma[1,2], Xuan Jin[1,2], Lei Chen[1,2], Ying Li[4], Jinqi Ma[4], Rong Ju[5], Jing Wei[1,6], Hongshan Ge[1,6], Qiuqin Tang[7]* and Wei Wu[1,2,3]*

1 State Key Laboratory of Reproductive Medicine and Offspring Health, Center for Global Health, Nanjing Medical University, Nanjing, China

2 Key Laboratory of Modern Toxicology of Ministry of Education, School of Public Health, Nanjing Medical University, Nanjing, China

3 Taizhou Clinical Medical College, Nanjing Medical University, Taizhou, China

4 The Affiliated Wuxi People's Hospital of Nanjing Medical University, Wuxi People's Hospital, Wuxi Medical Center, Nanjing Medical University, Wuxi, China

5 Department of Gynaecology and Obstetrics, Nanjing Jiangning Hospital Affiliated to Nanjing Medical University, Nanjing, China

6 Department of Obstetrics, The Affiliated Taizhou People's Hospital to Nanjing Medical University, Taizhou, China

7 Department of Obstetrics, Women's Hospital of Nanjing Medical University, Nanjing Maternity and Child Health Care Hospital, Nanjing, China

*Address all correspondence to: tqq19871004@126.com and wwu@njmu.edu.cn

References

[1] Giudice LC, Kao LC. Endometriosis. Lancet. 2004;**364**(9447):1789-1799

[2] Burney RO, Giudice LC. Pathogenesis and pathophysiology of endometriosis. Fertility and Sterility. 2012;**98**(3):511-519

[3] Koike E, Yasuda Y, Shiota M, et al. Exposure to ethinyl estradiol prenatally and/or after sexual maturity induces endometriotic and precancerous lesions in uteri and ovaries of mice. Congenital Anomalies (Kyoto). 2013;**53**(1):9-17

[4] Polak G, Banaszewska B, Filip M, et al. Environmental factors and endometriosis. International Journal of Environmental Research and Public Health. 2021;**18**(21):11025

[5] Giampaolino P, Della Corte L, Foreste V, et al. Dioxin and endometriosis: A new possible relation based on epigenetic theory. Gynecological Endocrinology. 2020;**36**(4):279-284

[6] Bruner-Tran KL, Ding T, Osteen KG. Dioxin and endometrial progesterone resistance. Seminars in Reproductive Medicine. 2010;**28**(1):59-68

[7] Pivonello C, Muscogiuri G, Nardone A, et al. Bisphenol A: An emerging threat to female fertility. Reproductive Biology and Endocrinology. 2020;**18**(1):22

[8] Chitakwa N, Alqudaimi M, Sultan M, et al. Plastic-related endocrine disrupting chemicals significantly related to the increased risk of estrogen-dependent diseases in women. Environmental Research. 2024;**252**(Pt. 2):118966

[9] Waddington CH. The epigenotype. International Journal of Epidemiology. 2012;**41**(1):10-13

[10] Zhang L, Lu Q, Chang C. Epigenetics in health and disease. Advances in Experimental Medicine and Biology. 2020;**1253**:3-55

[11] Guo SW. Epigenetics of endometriosis. Molecular Human Reproduction. 2009;**15**(10):587-607

[12] Koninckx PR, Ussia A, Adamyan L, et al. Pathogenesis of endometriosis: The genetic/epigenetic theory. Fertility and Sterility. 2019;**111**(2):327-340

[13] Gruber TM, Mechsner S. Pathogenesis of endometriosis: The origin of pain and subfertility. Cells. 2021;**10**(6):1381

[14] Farland LV, Degnan WJ, Harris HR, et al. Recreational and residential sun exposure and risk of endometriosis: A prospective cohort study. Human Reproduction. 2021;**36**(1):199-210

[15] Somigliana E, Viganò P, Abbiati A, et al. 'Here comes the sun': Pigmentary traits and sun habits in women with endometriosis. Human Reproduction. 2010;**25**(3):728-733

[16] Porpora MG, Ingelido AM, Di Domenico A, et al. Increased levels of polychlorobiphenyls in Italian women with endometriosis. Chemosphere. 2006;**63**(8):1361-1367

[17] Martínez-Zamora MA, Mattioli L, Parera J, et al. Increased levels of dioxin-like substances in adipose tissue in patients with deep infiltrating endometriosis. Human Reproduction. 2015;**30**(5):1059-1068

[18] Kim SH, Cho S, Ihm HJ, et al. Possible role of phthalate in the pathogenesis of endometriosis: In vitro,

animal, and human data. The Journal of Clinical Endocrinology and Metabolism. 2015;**100**(12):E1502-E1511

[19] Cobellis L, Latini G, De Felice C, et al. High plasma concentrations of di-(2-ethylhexyl)-phthalate in women with endometriosis. Human Reproduction. 2003;**18**(7):1512-1515

[20] Geens T, Aerts D, Berthot C, et al. A review of dietary and non-dietary exposure to bisphenol-A. Food and Chemical Toxicology. 2012;**50**(10):3725-3740

[21] Rashtian J, Chavkin DE, Merhi Z. Water and soil pollution as determinant of water and food quality/contamination and its impact on female fertility. Reproductive Biology and Endocrinology. 2019;**17**(1):5

[22] Rzymski P, Tomczyk K, Rzymski P, et al. Impact of heavy metals on the female reproductive system. Annals of Agricultural and Environmental Medicine. 2015;**22**(2):259-264

[23] Dutta S, Gorain B, Choudhury H, et al. Environmental and occupational exposure of metals and female reproductive health. Environmental Science and Pollution Research International. 2022;**29**(41):62067-62092

[24] Johnson MD, Kenney N, Stoica A, et al. Cadmium mimics the in vivo effects of estrogen in the uterus and mammary gland. Nature Medicine. 2003;**9**(8):1081-1084

[25] Jackson LW, Zullo MD, Goldberg JM. The association between heavy metals, endometriosis and uterine myomas among premenopausal women: National health and nutrition examination survey 1999-2002. Human Reproduction. 2008;**23**(3):679-687

[26] Human Microbiome Project Consortium. Structure, function and diversity of the healthy human microbiome. Nature. 2012;**486**(7402):207-214

[27] Kovács Z, Glover L, Reidy F, et al. Novel diagnostic options for endometriosis - Based on the glycome and microbiome. Journal of Advanced Research. 2021;**33**:167-181

[28] Ata B, Yildiz S, Turkgeldi E, et al. The endobiota study: Comparison of vaginal, cervical and gut microbiota between women with stage 3/4 endometriosis and healthy controls. Scientific Reports. 2019;**9**(1):2204

[29] Berkkanoglu M, Arici A. Immunology and endometriosis. American Journal of Reproductive Immunology. 2003;**50**(1):48-59

[30] Laschke MW, Menger MD. The gut microbiota: A puppet master in the pathogenesis of endometriosis? American Journal of Obstetrics and Gynecology. 2016;**215**(1):68.e1-68.e4

[31] Halis G, Arici A. Endometriosis and inflammation in infertility. Annals of the New York Academy of Sciences. 2004;**1034**:300-315

[32] Halme J, Becker S, Wing R. Accentuated cyclic activation of peritoneal macrophages in patients with endometriosis. American Journal of Obstetrics and Gynecology. 1984;**148**(1):85-90

[33] Wu M-H, Hsiao K-Y, Tsai S-J. Endometriosis and possible inflammation markers. Gynecology and Minimally Invasive Therapy. 2015;**4**(3):61-67

[34] Reis FM, Petraglia F, Taylor RN. Endometriosis: Hormone regulation and clinical consequences of chemotaxis and apoptosis. Human Reproduction Update. 2013;**19**(4):406-418

[35] Mohammed Rasheed HA, Hamid P. Inflammation to infertility: Panoramic view on endometriosis. Cureus. 2020;**12**(11):e11516

[36] Salliss ME, Farland LV, Mahnert ND, et al. The role of gut and genital microbiota and the estrobolome in endometriosis, infertility and chronic pelvic pain. Human Reproduction Update. 2021;**28**(1):92-131

[37] Tang F, Deng M, Xu C, et al. Unraveling the microbial puzzle: Exploring the intricate role of gut microbiota in endometriosis pathogenesis. Frontiers in Cellular and Infection Microbiology. 2024;**14**:1328419

[38] Baker JM, Al-Nakkash L, Herbst-Kralovetz MM. Estrogen-gut microbiome axis: Physiological and clinical implications. Maturitas. 2017;**103**:45-53

[39] Marino JL, Holt VL, Chen C, et al. Shift work, hCLOCK T3111C polymorphism, and endometriosis risk. Epidemiology. 2008;**19**(3):477-484

[40] Labyak S, Lava S, Turek F, et al. Effects of shiftwork on sleep and menstrual function in nurses. Health Care for Women International. 2002;**23**(6-7):703-714

[41] Parazzini F, Viganò P, Candiani M, et al. Diet and endometriosis risk: A literature review. Reproductive Biomedicine Online. 2013;**26**(4):323-336

[42] Nodler JL, Divasta AD, Vitonis AF, et al. Supplementation with vitamin D or ω-3 fatty acids in adolescent girls and young women with endometriosis (SAGE): A double-blind, randomized, placebo-controlled trial. The American Journal of Clinical Nutrition. 2020;**112**(1):229-236

[43] Grodstein F, Goldman MB, Ryan L, et al. Relation of female infertility to consumption of caffeinated beverages. American Journal of Epidemiology. 1993;**137**(12):1353-1360

[44] Mccarty M, Avery OT. Studies on the chemical nature of the substance inducing transformation of pneumococcal types: II. Effect of desoxyribonuclease on the biological activity of the transforming substance. The Journal of Experimental Medicine. 1946;**83**(2):89-96

[45] Griffith JS, Mahler HR. DNA ticketing theory of memory. Nature. 1969;**223**(5206):580-582

[46] Saxonov S, Berg P, Brutlag DL. A genome-wide analysis of CpG dinucleotides in the human genome distinguishes two distinct classes of promoters. Proceedings of the National Academy of Sciences of the United States of America. 2006;**103**(5):1412-1417

[47] Mohn F, Weber M, Rebhan M, et al. Lineage-specific polycomb targets and de novo DNA methylation define restriction and potential of neuronal progenitors. Molecular Cell. 2008;**30**(6):755-766

[48] Moore LD, Le T, Fan G. DNA methylation and its basic function. Neuropsychopharmacology. 2013;**38**(1):23-38

[49] Zondervan KT, Becker CM, Koga K, et al. Endometriosis. Nature Reviews. Disease Primers. 2018;**4**(1):9

[50] Arnal JF, Lenfant F, Metivier R, et al. Membrane and nuclear estrogen receptor alpha actions: From tissue specificity to medical implications. Physiological Reviews. 2017;**97**(3):1045-1087

[51] Dyson MT, Kakinuma T, Pavone ME, et al. Aberrant expression and

localization of deoxyribonucleic acid methyltransferase 3B in endometriotic stromal cells. Fertility and Sterility. 2015;**104**(4):953-963.e2

[52] Chantalat E, Valera MC, Vaysse C, et al. Estrogen receptors and endometriosis. International Journal of Molecular Sciences. 2020;**21**(8):2815

[53] Pellegrini C, Gori I, Achtari C, et al. The expression of estrogen receptors as well as GREB1, c-MYC, and cyclin D1, estrogen-regulated genes implicated in proliferation, is increased in peritoneal endometriosis. Fertility and Sterility. 2012;**98**(5):1200-1208

[54] Xue Q, Lin Z, Cheng YH, et al. Promoter methylation regulates estrogen receptor 2 in human endometrium and endometriosis. Biology of Reproduction. 2007;**77**(4):681-687

[55] Bulun SE, Utsunomiya H, Lin Z, et al. Steroidogenic factor-1 and endometriosis. Molecular and Cellular Endocrinology. 2009;**300**(1-2):104-108

[56] Izawa M, Taniguchi F, Uegaki T, et al. Demethylation of a nonpromoter cytosine-phosphate-guanine island in the aromatase gene may cause the aberrant up-regulation in endometriotic tissues. Fertility and Sterility. 2011;**95**(1):33-39

[57] Wu Y, Strawn E, Basir Z, et al. Promoter hypermethylation of progesterone receptor isoform B (PR-B) in endometriosis. Epigenetics. 2006;**1**(2):106-111

[58] Riaz MA, Kary FL, Jensen A, et al. Long-term maintenance of viable human endometrial epithelial cells to analyze estrogen and progestin effects. Cells. 2024;**13**(10):811

[59] Hayashi A, Tanabe A, Kawabe S, et al. Dienogest increases the progesterone receptor isoform B/A ratio in patients with ovarian endometriosis. Journal of Ovarian Research. 2012;**5**(1):31

[60] Squatrito M, Vervier J, Bindels J, et al. Impaired fertility in adenomyosis: A murine model reveals endometrial receptivity and progesterone resistance imbalances. Reproduction. 2024;**167**(5):e240019

[61] Lei L, Xu X, Gong C, et al. Integrated analysis of genome-wide gene expression and DNA methylation profiles reveals candidate genes in ovary endometriosis. Frontiers in Endocrinology (Lausanne). 2023;**14**:1093683

[62] Zubrzycka A, Zubrzycki M, Perdas E, et al. Genetic, epigenetic, and steroidogenic modulation mechanisms in endometriosis. Journal of Clinical Medicine. 2020;**9**(5):1309

[63] Zhang Y, Sun Z, Jia J, et al. Overview of histone modification. Advances in Experimental Medicine and Biology. 2021;**1283**:1-16

[64] Monteiro JB, Colón-Díaz M, García M, et al. Endometriosis is characterized by a distinct pattern of histone 3 and histone 4 lysine modifications. Reproductive Sciences. 2014;**21**(3):305-318

[65] Nasu K, Kawano Y, Kai K, et al. Aberrant histone modification in endometriosis. Frontiers in Bioscience (Landmark Edition). 2014;**19**(8):1202-1214

[66] Krol J, Loedige I, Filipowicz W. The widespread regulation of microRNA biogenesis, function and decay. Nature Reviews. Genetics. 2010;**11**(9):597-610

[67] Zhou M, Fu J, Xiao L, et al. miR-196a overexpression activates the MEK/ERK signal and represses the progesterone

receptor and decidualization in eutopic endometrium from women with endometriosis. Human Reproduction. 2016;**31**(11):2598-2608

[68] Nazri HM, Greaves E, Quenby S, et al. The role of small extracellular vesicle-miRNAs in endometriosis. Human Reproduction. 2023;**38**(12):2296-2311

[69] Wang Y, Li Y, Yang Z, et al. Genome-wide microarray analysis of long non-coding RNAs in eutopic secretory endometrium with endometriosis. Cellular Physiology and Biochemistry. 2015;**37**(6):2231-2245

[70] Ferlita A, Battaglia R, Andronico F, et al. Non-coding RNAs in endometrial physiopathology. International Journal of Molecular Sciences. 2018;**19**(7):2120

[71] Smolarz B, Szyłło K, Romanowicz H. Endometriosis: Epidemiology, classification, pathogenesis, treatment and genetics (review of literature). International Journal of Molecular Sciences. 2021;**22**(19):10554

[72] Burney RO, Talbi S, Hamilton AE, et al. Gene expression analysis of endometrium reveals progesterone resistance and candidate susceptibility genes in women with endometriosis. Endocrinology. 2007;**148**(8):3814-3826

[73] Patel BG, Rudnicki M, Yu J, et al. Progesterone resistance in endometriosis: Origins, consequences and interventions. Acta Obstetricia et Gynecologica Scandinavica. 2017;**96**(6):623-632

[74] Al-Sabbagh M, Lam EW, Brosens JJ. Mechanisms of endometrial progesterone resistance. Molecular and Cellular Endocrinology. 2012;**358**(2):208-215

[75] Garcia E, Bouchard P, De Brux J, et al. Use of immunocytochemistry of progesterone and estrogen receptors for endometrial dating. The Journal of Clinical Endocrinology and Metabolism. 1988;**67**(1):80-87

[76] Lessey BA, Yeh I, Castelbaum AJ, et al. Endometrial progesterone receptors and markers of uterine receptivity in the window of implantation. Fertility and Sterility. 1996;**65**(3):477-483

[77] Attia GR, Zeitoun K, Edwards D, et al. Progesterone receptor isoform A but not B is expressed in endometriosis. The Journal of Clinical Endocrinology and Metabolism. 2000;**85**(8):2897-2902

[78] Lindsay TJ, Vitrikas KR. Evaluation and treatment of infertility. American Family Physician. 2015;**91**(5):308-314

[79] Verkauf BS. Incidence, symptoms, and signs of endometriosis in fertile and infertile women. The Journal of the Florida Medical Association. 1987;**74**(9):671-675

[80] Bonavina G, Taylor HS. Endometriosis-associated infertility: From pathophysiology to tailored treatment. Frontiers in Endocrinology (Lausanne). 2022;**13**:1020827

[81] Pembrey M, Saffery R, Bygren LO. Human transgenerational responses to early-life experience: Potential impact on development, health and biomedical research. Journal of Medical Genetics. 2014;**51**(9):563-572

[82] Gayon J. From Mendel to epigenetics: History of genetics. Comptes Rendus Biologies. 2016;**339**(7-8):225-230

[83] Klosin A, Casas E, Hidalgo-Carcedo C, et al. Transgenerational transmission of environmental information in *C. Elegans*. Science. 2017;**356**(6335):320-323

[84] Ge C, Ye J, Weber C, et al. The histone demethylase KDM6B regulates temperature-dependent sex determination in a turtle species. Science. 2018;**360**(6389):645-648

[85] Koninckx PR, Ussia A, Tahlak M, et al. Infection as a potential cofactor in the genetic-epigenetic pathophysiology of endometriosis: A systematic review. Facts, Views & Vision in ObGyn. 2019;**11**(3):209-216

[86] Barker DJ. The fetal and infant origins of adult disease. BMJ. 1990;**301**(6761):1111

[87] Moustafa S, Burn M, Mamillapalli R, et al. Accurate diagnosis of endometriosis using serum microRNAs. American Journal of Obstetrics and Gynecology. 2020;**223**(4):557.e1-557.e11

[88] Wang WT, Sun YM, Huang W, et al. Genome-wide long non-coding RNA analysis identified circulating LncRNAs as novel non-invasive diagnostic biomarkers for gynecological disease. Scientific Reports. 2016;**6**:23343

[89] Hirakawa T, Nasu K, Aoyagi Y, et al. ATM expression is attenuated by promoter hypermethylation in human ovarian endometriotic stromal cells. Molecular Human Reproduction. 2019;**25**(6):295-304